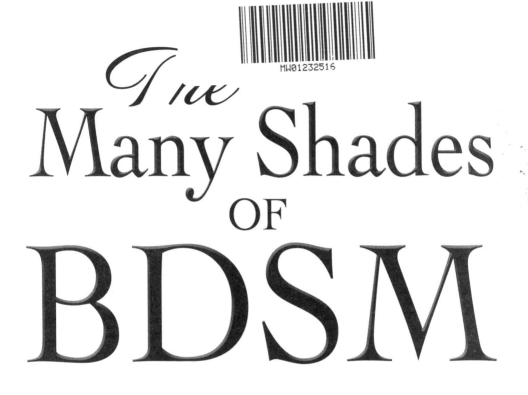

The
Many Shades
OF
BDSM

A Safe and **SCINTILLATING ENTRY** Into
the **ESCALATING PLEASURE** of BDSM

B. J. DEMPSEY

Author of *1,001 Sexcapades to Do If You Dare*

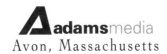
A**adams**media
Avon, Massachusetts

Published by
Adams Media, a division of F+W Media, Inc.
57 Littlefield Street, Avon, MA 02322. U.S.A.
www.adamsmedia.com

ISBN 10: 1-4405-5252-5
ISBN 13: 978-1-4405-5252-6
eISBN 10: 1-4405-5253-3
eISBN 13: 978-1-4405-5253-3

Printed in the United States of America.

10   9   8   7   6   5   4   3   2

Contains material adapted and abridged from *The Everything® Tantric Sex Book* by Bobbi Dempsey, copyright © 2007 by F+W Media, Inc., ISBN 10: 1-59869-326-3, ISBN 13: 978-1-59869-326-3; *1,001 Sexcapades to Do If You Dare* by Bobbi Dempsey, copyright © 2008 by F+W Media, Inc., ISBN 10: 1-59869-903-2; ISBN 13: 978-1-59869-903-6; and *The Everything® Great Sex Book, 2nd Edition* by Bobbi Dempsey, copyright © 2010, 2004 by F+W Media, Inc., ISBN 10: 1-4405-0148-3; ISBN 13: 978-1-4405-0148-7.

Readers are urged to take all appropriate precautions before undertaking any how-to task. Always read and follow instructions and safety warnings for all tools and materials, and call in a professional if the task stretches your abilities too far. Although every effort has been made to provide the best possible information in this book, neither the publisher nor the author are responsible for accidents, injuries, or damage incurred as a result of tasks undertaken by readers. This book is not a substitute for professional services.

Many of the designations used by manufacturers and sellers to distinguish their product are claimed as trademarks. Where those designations appear in this book and Adams Media was aware of a trademark claim, the designations have been printed with initial capital letters.

This book is available at quantity discounts for bulk purchases.
For information, please call 1-800-289-0963.

This is for all the lovers who want to unleash their wild side.

Acknowledgments

The author would like to thank Gina Panettieri of Talcott Notch Literary and Andrea Hakanson of Adams Media for their help with this project.

Contents

Introduction

Welcome, and thanks for joining me. By reading this book, you are taking the first step toward a new and exciting journey in your sexual adventures. Whether you are eager to jump into BDSM right this very minute with gusto or are just curious and want to explore the idea, you are motivated to add a spark to your sex life—and that is always a good thing! This shows you realize that your pleasure (and your partner's) is a priority, and you embrace the opportunity to try new things in order to share many new and wonderful intimate moments together.

Just by reading this book and taking other steps—even if they are baby steps—toward exploring more daring and risky sexual activities, you show that you are open to spicing up your physical relationship. That is a great step, as lots of thrilling and possibly earth-shattering moments can result from opening your mind to new intimate experiences.

You may have many reasons for exploring the world of BDSM. Maybe you fear that you have gotten in a rut or are heading in that direction. Or you may have had these secret yearnings and curiosities for a long time, yet held off because you were nervous or afraid—or just didn't know how to get started. Perhaps you have been fantasizing about being tied up, or getting spanked, or even serving as a sex slave—and now you want to see if the reality can match up to your X-rated visions.

It is also possible that you have suddenly been hearing a lot about it and are itching to see what all the fuss is about. BDSM has suddenly become trendy, which means you may have found yourself seeing and thinking about it much more than you ever did in the past. The fact that BDSM is hot right now can also make it seem a little more acceptable—and possibly a bit less scary. Maybe some of your friends are doing it—and raving about it—and you want to see just what is putting those naughty smiles on their faces.

Whatever your reason, I am glad you are taking this first step. BDSM can be a very exciting and enjoyable way to take your sex life in a thrilling new direction. It can allow you and your partner to share some unforgettable experiences, ones that quite possibly may take you to greater heights of pleasure than you have ever imagined. True, BDSM isn't for everyone, but you owe it to yourself to satisfy your burning curiosity (and growing desire) by at least giving it a try.

Think BDSM (at least parts of it) may be too wild or dangerous for you? No problem. The great thing about BDSM—and any sexual activity, really—is there are no ironclad rules. You can experiment and try things out, and then decide what works for you. If one thing sends shivers through your body (in a good way) and allows you to reach more powerful climaxes than ever before—well, obviously you will want to keep enjoying that experience. But if you try something and discover it isn't for you—well, at least you were brave enough to try, and now you know you can cross that activity off your list. Either way, you will probably have fun doing the research.

Most likely, you will find at least a few things that you really enjoy, and then you can tailor those specific things to your own individual tastes, making them as intense and wild (or not) as you like. You can also take the BDSM basics—spanking or restraints, for example—and put your own unique and personal spin on them, making the experience something completely personal for you and your partner. You can proceed at your own pace, taking whatever direction feels comfortable or exciting for you. Have fun blazing new trails!

You will probably discover some new things about yourself and your partner along the way. You just might surprise yourself by uncovering some powerful urges and strong turn-ons you never even knew you had—which may make you wish you had done this a long time ago! And if you are a little bit nervous about trying BDSM, you will enjoy a sense of accomplishment once you conquer this new territory. You will likely feel empowered at your new boldness, and will revel in your role as a fierce sex god or goddess.

Whether you take the dominant or submissive role, you may find that a BDSM arrangement frees you to shed your inhibitions and explore your sexuality in a way you have never done before. That can pave the way to many wonderful new experiences and sensations.

Now that you have taken the first step, keep going! The information and tips in this book should help guide you on your way, and I hope to encourage you to proceed with gusto. Be bold and daring—you will be glad you did!

Chances are, you will discover some new tricks that add some hot sparks to your sex life. This will obviously improve your physical relationship, but can also help strengthen or renew your emotional bond. You will enjoy a new sort of intimate connection with your partner, and the two of you will benefit from exploring this shared adventure together.

So what are you waiting for? Lots of exciting new experiences lie ahead.

Enjoy the journey!

Chapter 1

An Introduction Into BDSM

"Everything in the world is about sex except sex. Sex is about power."

—Oscar Wilde

The world of BDSM is seductive, enticing, exciting, and a bit dangerous —which is why it's so much fun. If you've never incorporated a little B&D or S&M into your sex life, get ready to be blown away. It's about control—having all of it or losing it—and power, reward and punishment, and pure ecstasy. The acronym BDSM stands for Bondage, Discipline, and SadoMasochism. (Sometimes the initials also stand for dominant and submissive.) These practices are meant to be fun, stimulating, and a part of sexual play between consensual partners.

BDSM can take many different forms, from incorporating very casual and occasional mild forms of discipline (such as light spanking) to a much more formal and serious arrangement, which may include a fully stocked playroom and pieces of BDSM equipment and toys—we'll talk about these later.

If you are new to the idea of BDSM, you may be feeling intimidated, clueless, or confused. Perhaps you're wondering how to get started. That is completely normal. You don't have to do anything you are not comfortable with. The best advice for a beginner is: relax. You are probably building this up to be a huge, overwhelming, and scary vision in your head, which will only cause you—and perhaps your partner—lots of needless anxiety.

As with anything else in a romantic relationship, BDSM varies greatly depending on personal preference. You can take it as slowly as you like, and figure out along the way just what works best for the two of you as a couple. Bonus: the adventure of trying new things and exploring your turn-ons can be a lot of fun and might take your ordinary sex routine to another mind-blowing level!

B&D (Bondage and Dominance/Discipline)

The "B" and "D" parts of BDSM refer to bondage and dominance or discipline. This can involve a wide range of activities, along a spectrum that ranges from tame to intense. Many people first get started in BDSM through some mild bondage or discipline activities. This is often accidental or unplanned. You may use a scarf to tie up a partner on a whim. Or your partner might get caught up in a passionate moment and give you a few playful spanks. In this case, you might discover (perhaps to your complete surprise) that you enjoy the experience—both the physical sensation and the idea of adding some "rough" play to your sex life. You may soon find yourself making this type of play a regular part of your bedroom routine. You might also decide to delve further into the world of bondage and discipline and explore other types of BDSM activities.

Bondage involves being tied up or restrained in some way. This can cause several titillating feelings—physically, emotionally, and mentally. Not only will you have the new physical feelings caused by being restrained, you will also experience the excitement of being at the mercy of someone else's control.

Then there is the element of teasing and delayed gratification. When you are restrained in some way, you cannot move parts of your body and probably cannot touch yourself and/or your partner, which can build the anticipation and greatly heighten your sexual arousal. This can add a major thrill to even the most "routine" sexual encounter.

These types of activities require a considerable amount of trust between you and your partner. Many people say this creates a new level

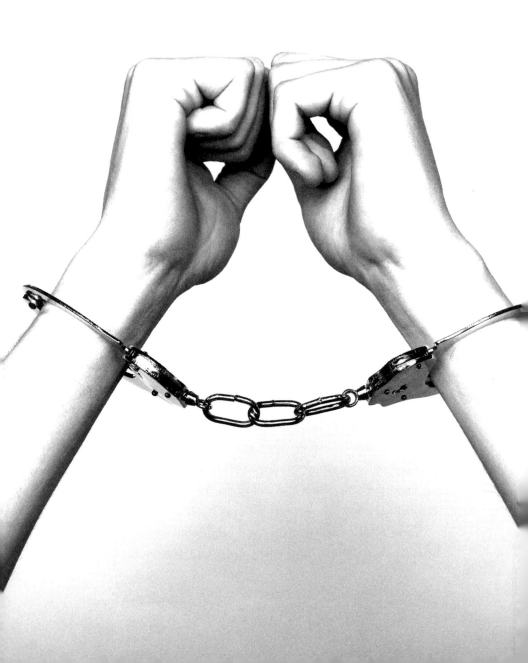

of intimacy and helps them develop a stronger bond and a more sensual connection as a couple.

S&M (Sadomasochism)

The term "sadomasochism" can be shocking or intimidating to a lot of people. This is partly because it is a bit misunderstood, and there are lots of misconceptions and stereotypes when it comes to sexual activities in this area. The term refers to deriving sexual pleasure from the pain experienced by you or others.

Many people mistakenly assume that S&M involves forcing other people to do something against their will or perhaps even torturing them. And although that may have been true of the sexual practice in some cultures and historical periods (and even perhaps sometimes in the current day), that's not what we are talking about here. We are dealing with the idea of sadomasochism as part of a BDSM lifestyle that is consensual and pleasurable for all parties involved.

For many people, the word sadomasochism conjures up visions of dark dungeons or whips and chains. These certainly do qualify as part of the sadomasochist realm, however, lots of other activities are more "beginner friendly" or don't require quite such a level of commitment (or bravery, depending on how you look at it). For example, you may want to ease your way into this form of sex play with some mild spanking or swats with a relatively soft paddle.

Of course, sadomasochism can run the gamut, all the way up to the other end of the spectrum—say, flogging or even activities involving

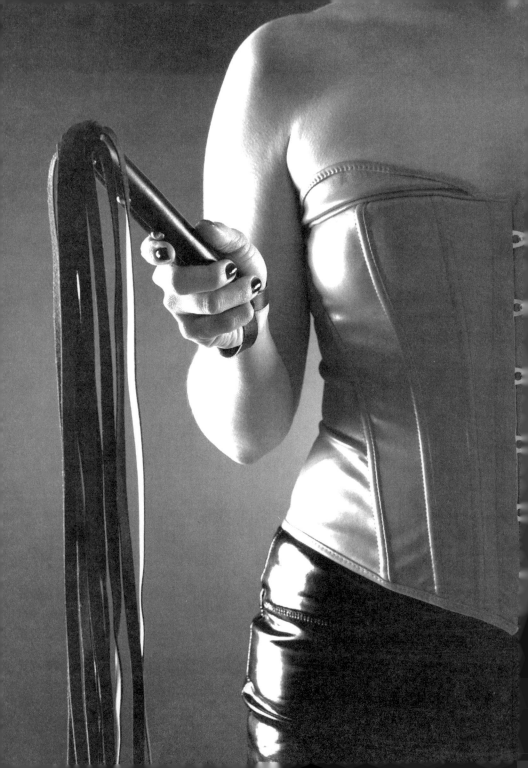

fire, hot wax, or similarly risky elements. These types of "hardcore" S&M activities are less common and usually aren't the first choice for casual experimenters or beginners.

Again, this is a matter of personal preference and your comfort level. Some people discover they are naturals when it comes to S&M, and they quickly want to dive right into the more intense practices. Part of the excitement of BDSM (and sex in general) comes from exploring your turn-ons and possibly discovering that you get really excited by something you might never have expected. This can be even more exciting when you help your partner bring out some of her hidden turn-ons. You never know where or when that thrill may pop up. Perhaps a week after you and your partner take your first baby steps into BDSM, he will suddenly start begging you to tie him up or let him put you in a spreader bar.

Keep an open mind and don't assume you know all of your own (or your partner's) pleasure triggers. Even if you are only mildly curious, it is probably worth trying something at least once just to see if you like it. You might be surprised with a naughty new playroom trick.

Dominants

In a BDSM situation involving two people, one must play the role of the dominant partner. A dominant or "dom" gives the orders and sets the rules, within the limits of a contract or agreement, if one has been established. Obviously, the dominant gets excited by being in control and inflicting pain (or perhaps simulated pain) on his or her partner. The dom likes to be the boss, and enjoys having power over the other person.

People often find that they have a natural tendency toward being a dominant or submissive—although it isn't uncommon for them to switch roles as an occasional temporary experiment, or even as a permanent change over time. Sometimes a person who was first initiated into BDSM as a submissive will later go on to become a dominant. And then, of course, the roles can evolve and change again.

It may seem as if a certain personality type would be more likely to play the dominant role. You might assume that this person is the bossy type, possibly a control freak—and that is often true. However, sometimes it's the opposite—someone who tends to be more mild-mannered in her everyday life will suddenly transform into a dominating personality behind closed doors. Along the same lines, if you are forced to take orders in your professional life (or even certain aspects of your personal life), you may really get off on unleashing your bossy side in the bedroom.

If you are first exploring BDSM and find that being in control excites you, you might be a little bit reluctant to show your dominant side—or even to acknowledge this role turns you on. There could be several reasons for this. If, as described above, you are normally the one who takes orders, the idea of being the one calling the shots may be intimidating or seem unnatural.

You might struggle with the idea of inflicting pain or embarrassment on another person. This is something you might just need to get used to over time. But this is also where a detailed contract—and lots

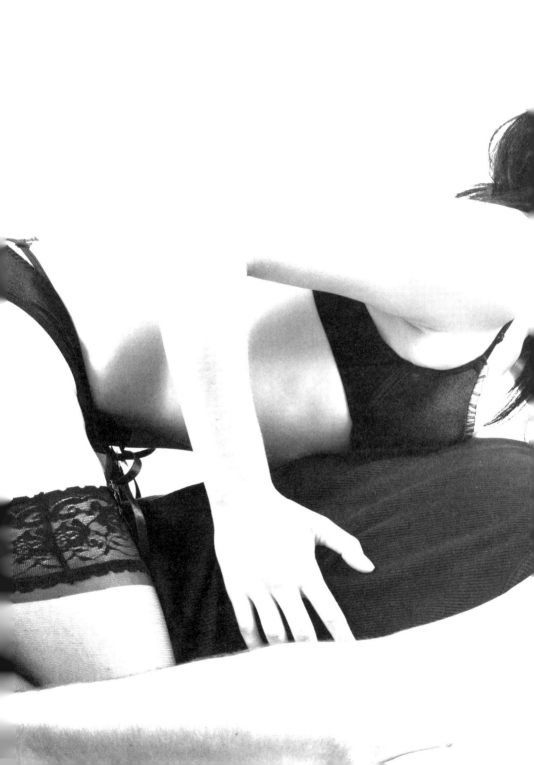

of open communication—can be so valuable. It is important to establish clear rules and boundaries. You want to know that you are only inflicting "good" pain or embarrassment on your partner—meaning, the type that he or she is okay with and finds exciting as a submissive.

The cardinal rule in this situation is that all activities must be consensual and both parties must agree. Knowing that you are only doing things that turn your partner on will probably help ease your mind and allow you to become more comfortable in a dominant role.

It can also help to look at this as if you are playing a role—which of course you are. Sex play is a game, and you are playing your part. You may even look at it as acting, just like any other sort of role-playing or acting out of a fantasy.

As a dominant, it is your responsibility to respect your submissive and adhere to the rules and boundaries you've both agreed to. If you disregard those boundaries or force the submissive to do something he doesn't want to do, you are breaking the trust that is essential for this type of relationship. On the other hand, you also have a sort of responsibility to hold up your end of the bargain by providing him with a thrilling experience. So if your submissive gets excited by you acting rough or putting on a show of "forcing" him to do something, then by all means do it with gusto. For example, if you realize that your submissive gets hot when you curse at her or "force" yourself on her, you may want to take a strong approach in doing those things. This part of the experience will often evolve gradually over time as you and your partner become more comfortable with your roles and explore your individual turn-ons.

Submissives

As a submissive, you are the one in the less powerful role—at least on the surface. Often the submissive has more power than she thinks. The submissive has power when it comes to establishing the ground rules and negotiating the contract (if you choose to use one).

As is true of a dominant, the submissive is not necessarily someone who seems to have an obviously submissive personality. There are many stories of people in powerful positions in the professional world who like to be dominated behind closed doors. For these people, who are constantly forced to give orders and make important decisions all day long, the idea of being ordered around can be very exciting.

The main role of a submissive is to relinquish all control. You might find it takes you a little while to become totally comfortable with this, especially if you tend to like being the powerful one who gives all the orders. In this case, you might need to ease into this role and allow yourself to be open to loosening up, releasing your inhibitions, and letting yourself just enjoy the physical (and mental) sensations of being under someone else's control.

Just because you are the one in the submissive role does not mean you don't have any control or say in what happens in your BDSM play. Just the opposite—it is important that you play an active role in setting up the arrangement and establishing rules and boundaries.

It is vital that you trust your partner and feel your partner respects you and will adhere to the rules you have both agreed to. If you are not quite sure you have that level of trust yet, be honest with your partner—and yourself. You need more time to reach that point. Give your

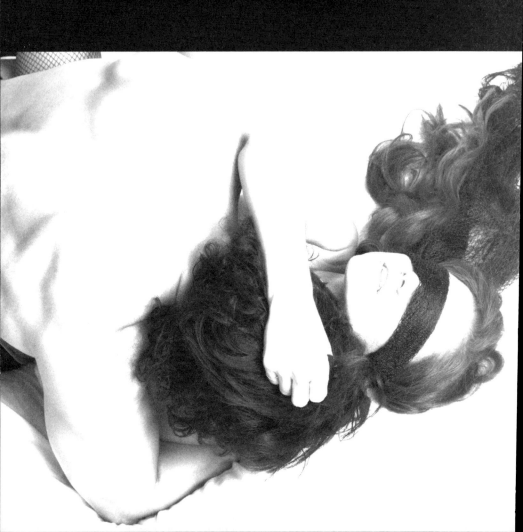

partner guidance as to what he or she can do to help you feel more comfortable and to establish that level of trust.

The role of a submissive can take many forms. You may simply be the one who submits to your partner's wishes and commands. From a physical and logistical standpoint, you are probably the one who will usually be restrained and/or disciplined. In more intense BDSM relationships, you may actually play the role of a sex slave. This can involve anything from wearing a leash and collar to perhaps acting like a servant and attending to your partner's daily personal needs, maybe even doing your partner's household chores.

Safe Is Sexy

Even though you may be the submissive one, you still have rights. You should never feel you have no choice but to do whatever your partner wants, regardless of whether you like it or not. You always have the right to say no. Your partner should never force you to do something you don't want to do. If this happens, you may need to reevaluate the relationship and consider whether you want to make some changes.

Switching

As we said earlier, you should not feel you are "locked in" to any one role. Granted, some people seem to be destined for one role or the other. Maybe you're sure you are a born dominator or a natural submissive.

But it is not uncommon for people to switch roles—in some cases, fairly often. This frequently happens with a change of partner. You may find that you were the submissive with your former partner, but have taken the dominant role with your current partner—perhaps because that person is more comfortable being the submissive.

Then again, you may find yourself switching roles even with the same partner. This can happen over time or it can be part of your ongoing routine. Some couples like to take turns switching roles. This may work well if both partners are turned on by being both the dominant and the submissive. By rotating roles, each partner gets to enjoy the thrilling aspects of each role. As a bonus, each has better insight and understanding into what it is like to be in the other role, which may help both people be more intuitive and attentive to what turns them on when they are in that role.

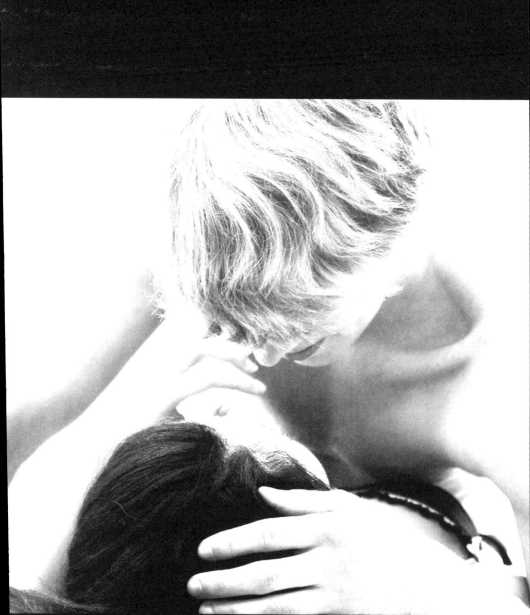

Chapter 2

Letting Go: Getting Comfortable with Being Bad

"Oh, the sweetness of giving in, of full surrender."

—Sebastian Faulks, *Engleby*

Taking a new step in your sex life—or in life in general—can require some courage. Trying new things can be scary. This can be especially true when it comes to our intimate activities, because these activities often require us not only to try new things physically, but also to expose ourselves emotionally and mentally. We may need to be more vulnerable and trusting than we have been in the past, and that can cause us to wrestle with hesitations and doubts.

The idea of "being bad" can also conjure up some negative messages we may have gotten about sex when we were growing up. This is especially common for women. As young girls, we may have been told that "good girls" don't do certain things. Breaking out of our shells, sexually speaking, can mean facing some deeply ingrained (mistaken) beliefs and misconceptions we may have about sex. For many people, just trying a position other than the standard missionary rut can seem like a big step, so it is only natural that the idea of BDSM may take some getting used to. Don't be surprised if you need to evaluate your whole way of thinking about sex and become comfortable with the idea of BDSM before you ever reach the point of trying it out in the bedroom or playroom.

But remember, there is nothing "bad" about getting physical pleasure from a sexual relationship with someone with whom you have a loving bond, someone whom you care about and have fun with. Fun activities between consenting adults are nothing to be ashamed of—and, by the way, they're also your own private business, so don't be concerned about what someone else may think.

Once you become comfortable with the idea of more daring sexual games, the next step is to actually try out some new moves in the bedroom. You may have to start slowly until you conquer your nerves and begin to relax. Fortunately, this isn't a race. You don't have to follow a timetable. You can "tiptoe" your way into this at whatever pace feels comfortable and pleasurable.

Now, with that out of the way, let's discuss some ways to get started so you can begin enjoying the fun. Because, as you will likely soon discover, being bad can feel oh so good!

Getting Your Partner Into It

Getting yourself to the point of being comfortable with BDSM is one thing. Getting your partner onboard with the idea is a whole other project. First, you will have to address (and possibly overcome) the same issues you may have faced yourself when first contemplating this new direction in your sexual play. You may need to help your partner, possibly guiding her through the same obstacles and inner conflicts you encountered.

Safe Is Sexy

Keep in mind the cardinal rule: You never want to pressure your partner or make your partner feel like you are judging him. You don't want to seem like you are criticizing her or making fun of her "hang-ups." Depending upon your partner's background and attitudes toward sex, she may have more issues to work through, and may need more time to become comfortable enough to try any sort of BDSM activities. It is important to use a light, no-pressure approach.

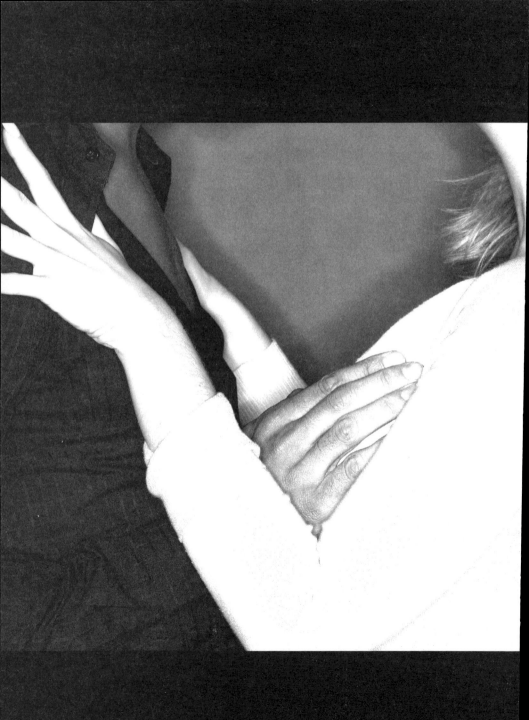

In addition to these common challenges and obstacles, you will also need to consider some other potential pitfalls when trying to get your partner onboard with the idea of BDSM bedroom fun. The following tips can help you avoid sabotaging your pro-BDSM campaign.

Focus on the Positive

It is critical that you focus on the positives in this situation. Be upbeat—like a sexual cheerleader. Stress the upsides, as in how these new additions to your sexual repertoire can add a new level of spice to your already great sexual relationship. You never want to say (or even imply) that your current relationship is lacking or that you are unsatisfied, even if that may actually be the case. Doing so will only make your partner feel bad and cause him to wonder if you have been secretly unhappy with your relationship for some time and have just been pretending to enjoy yourself when the two of you hit the sheets. This will have a negative impact on your partner's view toward your sexual relationship, and will probably make it even tougher to get him enthused about trying something new.

You also want to frame it in such a way that emphasizes its mutual benefits. BDSM should be something both of you will really enjoy, so don't only talk about your own turn-ons. Suggest a few new things in the BDSM realm that you think your partner might enjoy. If you can describe the scene in a sexy and vivid way, you might even get your lover so hot she will be eager to try out these new games with you.

Don't Seem Too Knowledgeable

This is one of those relationship situations that requires some discretion and diplomacy. You do not want to seem like you are the world's preeminent expert in BDSM. If you and your partner have never explored this type of sexual activity before and you suddenly display a wealth of knowledge on the topic, your partner will probably jump to one of two conclusions: either you had a wild past you have been hiding up until now, or (even worse) you've been cheating and have learned new tricks with another partner on the side.

To avoid these unpleasant scenarios from popping into your partner's head, the best approach is to frame this as something you have been curious about and possibly have even researched a little bit online (or by reading books, such as this one), and would like to start exploring together as a couple. Another tactic that might help you broach the topic in a nonthreatening way is to watch an X-rated movie that involves some scenes of BDSM activities portrayed in a sexy way. If you feel your partner might be scared off by anything too intense, look for films with scenes of relatively mild BDSM moves. You can then make it obvious to your partner that watching this is turning you on. With any luck, she may take the lead in starting a discussion about whether you two should try some similar moves in real life. If not, casually initiate the discussion yourself.

Save the Scary Stuff for Later

You want to gently warm your partner up to the idea of engaging in BDSM play with you. Start mild and work your way up to wild. If you start throwing around terms like clamps and gags right off the bat, you might cause your lover to run in fear. Instead, wait until you have warmed him up by showing him how much fun you two can have with some milder tactics such as spanking, and then gradually work your way up to the more serious stuff.

Flirtation and Teasing

When first introducing any new addition to your bedroom bag of tricks, your initial approach can make or break you. This is especially true in the case of BDSM activities, which can be unfamiliar or intimidating to many people (including, perhaps, your partner). Even though you might be chomping at the bit to show your submissive side or are drooling at the idea of tying your partner up, you do not want to come on too strong at this stage. You run the risk of scaring your partner off of the idea, or making him nervous that he may not be able to keep up or match your enthusiasm.

You also want to avoid putting too much pressure on yourself or your partner. As with anything new, you may stumble a bit or have a few awkward encounters when you first start. This is natural and to be expected. You might find that your first few attempts at BDSM play lead you to some unintentional funny experiences as you try to figure out what to do or how to work some of your new toys. Be prepared for this, and just roll with it. Although these moments may not be the hot and wild sexual romps you may have envisioned, some of the most enjoyable bedroom moments are the ones that make us laugh. If you have a good attitude and a sense of humor—both of which are essential in general for a satisfying and positive sexual relationship—you can have fun with these "blooper" moments, even if they didn't go the way you planned.

One way to start off in the right direction is to emphasize the flirtation aspect of the situation. Take your time in building the sexual tension, making the most of the opportunity to lavishly and sensually seduce your partner. By proceeding very slowly, you can build the anticipation and bring your partner to a point of peak excitement. If you play your cards right and do a good job with your flirting, you might find that he is begging you to tie him up, spank him, or engage in some other BDSM play.

By enjoying the flirting and the buildup process, you take some of the pressure off the "main event" itself and make it more likely that your partner will be hot and bothered and ready to play.

Kinky Tip

Nervous about your ability to tease or flirt with your partner as part of your BDSM buildup? Or just not sure where to start? Make a game of it by trying to work in certain keywords. For example, see if you can come up with a creative and/or sexy way to work the word "whip" into a seductive come-on. Or see how many synonyms for "punishment" you can come up with and use in a seemingly innocent conversation.

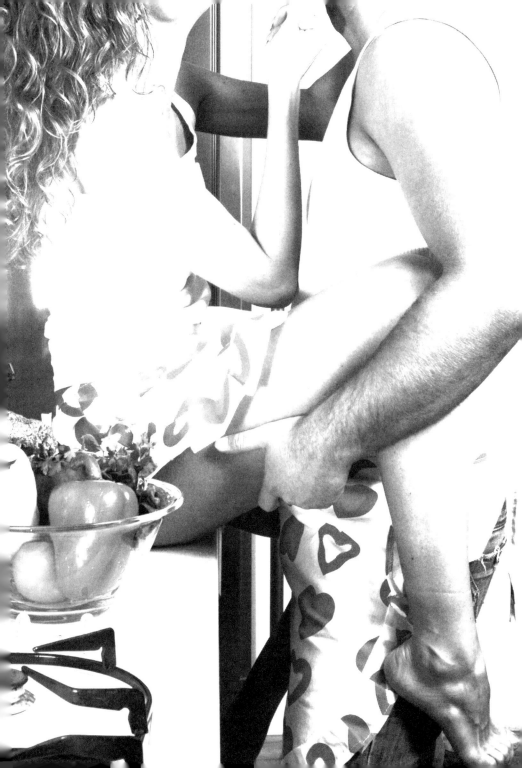

Teasing can also be an effective strategy. When used along with flirting, teasing can really help get your partner excited and eager to try some new tricks. You can seductively play with your partner's necktie with a knowing and naughty look, and perhaps even whisper a little hint of what naughty things you would like to do to him with it. Or drop a few comments about how he has been a "bad boy" and could really use some discipline—and you know exactly what punishment he needs.

You may even be able to use your insider knowledge of your partner's secret turn-ons to make your teasing more effective. Get creative, and be as graphic and/or descriptive as you can pull off comfortably. Make this as tempting and enticing as possible for your partner.

Introducing Kink Into Your Sex Life

If your sex life has been relatively tame up until this point, you may have mixed feelings about stepping up the kinky quotient of your sexual activities. As already discussed, taking this kind of step can be scary, making you feel anxious and nervous. You may also worry that you might seem like a "freak" or a sexual deviate.

Again, this is why it is so important to take baby steps and proceed at your own pace. You don't want to rush yourself or your partner into this, or you run the risk of being overwhelmed or freaked out, which may scare you off the idea of BDSM before you even give it a fair chance.

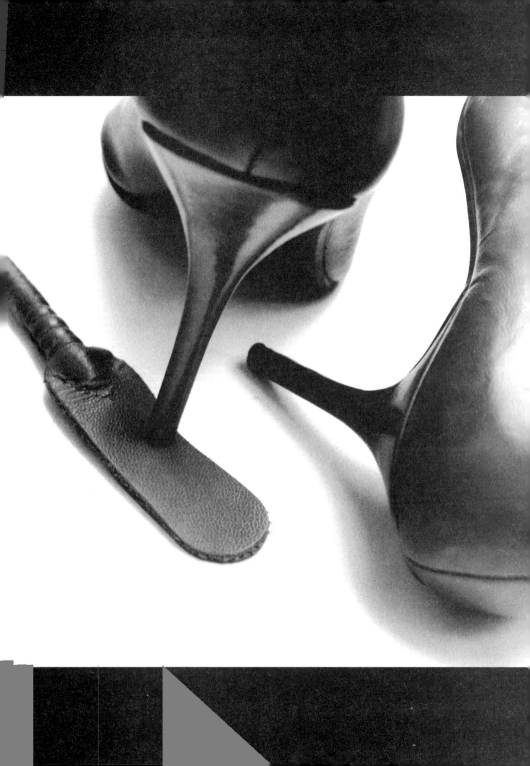

One thing that can help is to adjust your mindset. Rather than thinking of "kinky" as weird or freaky, think of it as another word for sexy.

Another trick: it can be fun to pretend you are playing a role. Instead of a meek and mild secretary (or whatever you are in real life), you are now going to be a fierce and fearless sexual tigress. Rather than being timid about your new kinky adventures, you will embrace your kinky side and show it off proudly.

Proceeding at the Right Pace

As in most things, when it comes to exploring the world of BDSM, timing is everything. This goes for not just the initial entry into "kink," but also to the progress of your journey along the way to BDSM ecstasy.

You do not want to push things along at such a fast pace that your partner feels rushed or pressured. This will likely backfire and make your partner even less eager to get onboard the BDSM bandwagon. Plus, it may cause tension in your relationship if your partner feels you are rushing her or trying to coerce her into doing something before she is fully ready.

Even if you are the one initiating this step into BDSM, it is possible to move too quickly for your own comfort, as well. Be careful not to get so caught up in the exciting idea of the thrill of BDSM that you rush into things before you are ready. This can leave you suddenly feeling overwhelmed or unprepared, or cause some awkward and

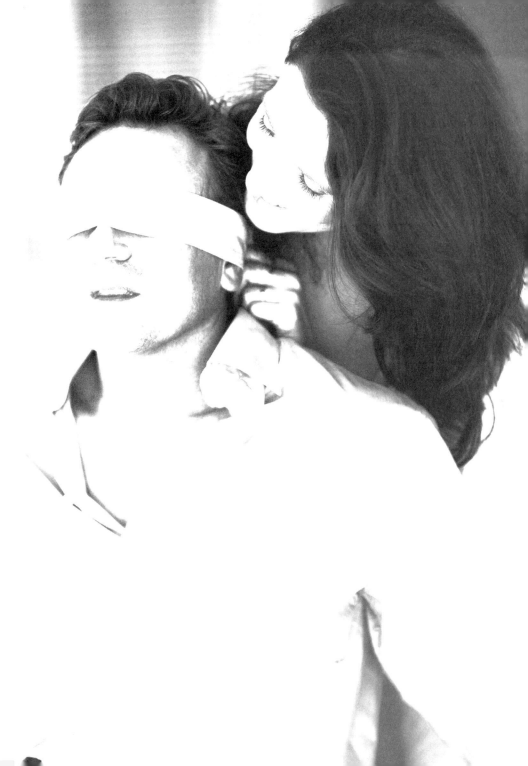

embarrassing moments at a time when you may have already passed the point of no return.

Rushing can also deprive you and your partner of the delicious buildup—which, as we all know, can be half the thrill of any sexual encounter. The teasing, anticipation, and rising excitement are all important elements in a scintillating sexual experience—and you don't want to miss out on any of it. True, the climax may be the ultimate goal, but don't overlook the many pleasurable peaks in the journey along the way to that end.

It is important to move slowly—but rather than viewing this as holding yourself back, look at it as a way to give yourself and your partner a chance to savor each step of the process. Think of it like enjoying a delightfully decadent meal for the first time. Luxuriate in the sensation and pleasure of every tiny little bite, letting your tongue caress every morsel and allowing all of your senses to revel in this exciting new experience.

If you are having trouble resisting the urge to speed right through to the hardcore BDSM big-time (possibly before either or both of you are ready), think of it as a game with many quests or levels along the way. Imagine that you earn a badge or award for each level you finish completely and thoroughly—perhaps when you "master" it after a certain period of time. Come up with imaginary or even real rewards that you and your partner can earn for completing each step or reaching "expert level" at each particular skill.

This approach will help you slow down and enjoy the ride without being too preoccupied with racing to get to a specific destination.

Safe Is Sexy

It can be easy to get so caught up in your own excitement when enjoying your BDSM playtime that you don't pay as much attention to your partner's comfort level as you should. It's a good idea to do a periodic "status check" and ask your partner how he feels about your new activities, just to make sure you are both on the same page.

Reaching Your Limit (and Pushing Your Boundaries)

At some point, you may find you have gone as far in the BDSM journey as you and/or your partner are comfortable with. This may be because you encounter several of your "hard limits" or simply because you are not interested in proceeding with anything more intense. Or maybe you have already found your favorite new playtime activities and don't feel the need to push yourselves into doing anything else.

Regardless of the reason, it's important to recognize when you have reached your limit. You must then decide what you want to do next. If you are satisfied with the skills you have mastered and want to stick with those activities, that's fine. The important thing is that you both feel content with that decision. If one of you really has the urge to continue on to try more risky things, he may feel resentful if you don't feel the same way—which may be something you need to address and discuss.

Then again, you may decide (and again, this is something you both must agree on) to push your boundaries and go a little bit further,

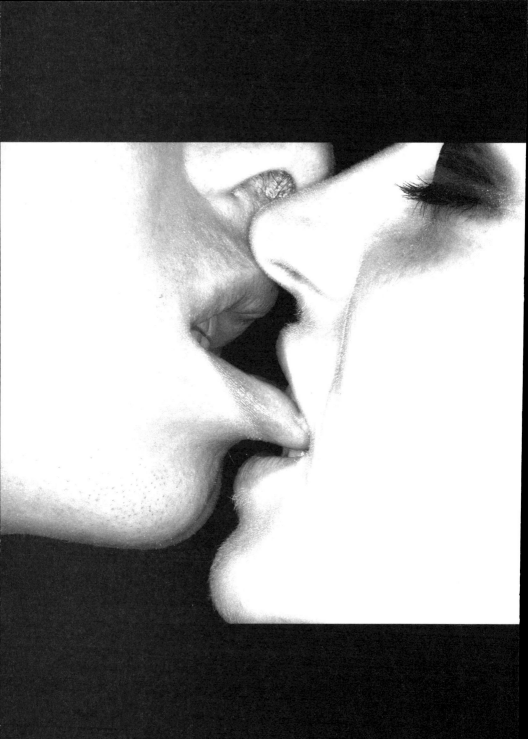

despite the fact that you might be unsure or nervous. For many people, part of the excitement of BDSM is the idea of trying things that are scary, dangerous, or perhaps even painful (in a good way). In that case, hitting this point can seem like an exciting challenge—a way for you to face and overcome your inhibitions or fears.

Pushing your boundaries and stepping outside your comfort zone can give you a powerful rush. You might find this to be intoxicating— and you also might feel a sense of pride and accomplishment from daring to do things you might not have thought you were capable of.

Bottom line: there is no one "right" way to handle the decision of where to go once you have reached this point in your playtime journey.

So how do you know if you have truly reached your limit or simply come to a point where the road gets a little more bumpy, yet adventurous? That's an individual decision you and your partner must address yourselves, together.

Chapter 3

Talk to Me: Establishing Rules and Trust

"The best way to find out if you can trust somebody is to trust them."

—Ernest Hemingway

Trust is an important part of any relationship. Many people would say it is the most important thing—or at least, right up there near the top of the list. Trust issues can kill any relationship—whether it is with a coworker, friend, family member, or romantic partner. So it goes without saying that you need to have a strong foundation of trust for a loving relationship—especially one that involves sexual intimacy.

When you take that sexual relationship to the next level and add BDSM to the mix, trust takes on an additional significance. Not only are you now exposing yourself more sexually and emotionally, leaving yourself more vulnerable, but in some cases you also may be putting your physical safety in the hands of another person. That person may have the ability to hurt you not just emotionally, but physically, as well. This requires a deep level of mutual trust, as each of you is trusting the other with your body and its well-being.

If you already have some trust issues in your relationship, or if your relationship is on shaky ground in any way that makes it difficult for you to completely trust your partner, this may not be the best time for you to consider adding BDSM activities to your sex life. It is probably a good idea to work on the other issues first and strengthen your relationship, so that you can approach BDSM from a place of total trust when you are ready.

Next, you need to establish a set of rules. Yes, we know you probably don't like rules. Many of us don't. In fact, we may take pride in being rule-breakers or "playing by our own rules." And, generally speaking, breaking some rules can add an extra element of sexiness and possibly even danger to your bedroom antics. But when introducing BDSM to your sex life, this is one situation where rules are not only a good thing—they are absolutely essential.

Rules define your limits and boundaries, so that neither of you feels pressured or obligated to do something you don't like. Establishing guidelines by spelling them out in a detailed set of rules from the beginning will help avoid many awkward or uncomfortable moments later, and will help both of you feel more relaxed and secure about going forward with your exploration of BDSM.

 Kinky Tip

To make the rule-making process seem more like fun and less like school, try coming up with some fun rules that can help heighten your anticipation or make the experience more sensual. For example, you might want to make a rule that your partner cannot touch you while you are teasing or pleasuring her. This will drive her crazy!

Take your time creating and refining your rules. Put some thought into them, and make sure to discuss them together as a couple. The goal is to come up with a set of rules that makes both of you feel comfortable.

Consent and Personal Safety

The first and possibly most important rules you need to address and discuss are those involving consent and personal safety. Consent is a big deal, because neither partner should be forced—or even have the feeling of being forced—to do something he or she does not want to do.

Clearly outline the issues of consent, spelling out exactly what each person consents to and does not consent to. Be specific as to what exactly constitutes consent. Can you agree to something in the heat of the moment, or do you have to consent beforehand, when you might be thinking more clearly? And what happens if someone initially consents to an activity, but then later changes his mind?

It may feel a bit too formal to write down a list of official rules, but this can be a valuable tool in helping to ensure neither of you feels you have been coerced into doing something. This prevents tension and resentment—things that can really kill your BDSM buzz.

Safe Is Sexy

A helpful tactic to use when you are first starting out with new BDSM activities is to clearly tell your partner what you are about to do. Yes, surprises can be sexy later on. But at this point when you are establishing trust, explaining—in a tantalizing and enticing way—what you're going to do can help make your partner feel more comfortable. It also gives her a chance to object, should you inadvertently start to approach one of her soft or hard limits.

Personal safety is another top priority. Carefully consider any activities or situations you will be engaging in, and think about any potential risks to your personal safety—then take all necessary steps

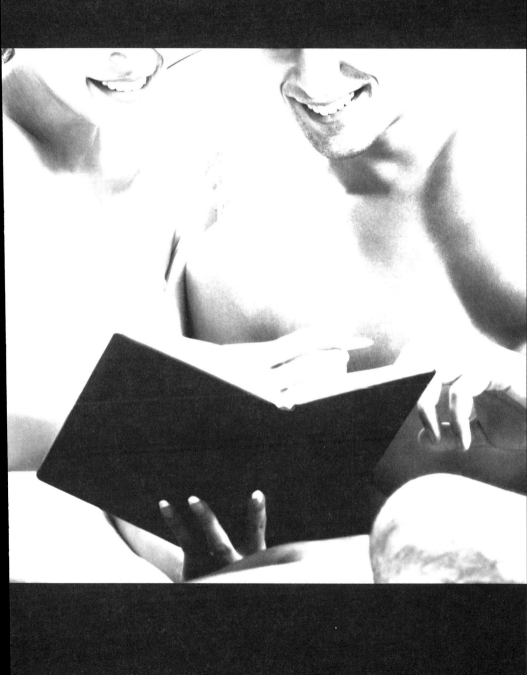

to eliminate the risk of personal injury. Obviously, this is a subjective thing, as many BDSM activities do, by definition, involve some degree of pain. But there should not be the danger of serious or permanent injury. Keep in mind that in many cases the *idea* of some risk or danger is the turn-on—not the reality of getting hurt.

It is almost impossible to be too careful when it comes to ensuring your personal safety, especially with BDSM activities that involve restraints, whips, or other equipment. This is not a situation in which you want to leave anything to chance. Nothing will kill a passionate mood quicker than a close call with a painful or serious injury.

Discussing Emotions and Fears

As many of us discover, our physical pleasure is closely connected to our emotions—even if we have (or try to have) a casual, no-strings-attached arrangement. In order to establish trust, have a frank and open discussion with your partner about your feelings and how they relate to your intimate relationships and turn-ons. Before you can do this, though, you may need to do some soul searching and deep inner reflection on your own. Often we do not even recognize or acknowledge our emotional motivations or triggers until we dig fairly deep.

We all have our own individual emotional "baggage." This is often tied to our backgrounds, experiences, and the messages we've gotten from the media and our families. We may not even realize we have certain feelings about love, sex, and other relationship issues until something triggers an emotional reaction and causes buried feelings to come to the surface.

Be alert for your own instinctive triggers and emotional reactions that could give you a clue as to how your feelings may come into play in your sexual encounters—especially when adding a new element such as BDSM to your sex life. For example, if you notice that you have a tendency to become upset or feel hurt if your partner snaps at you or uses a serious tone of voice, you will want to make sure you are prepared for the emotional fallout that may result from him as a dominant ordering you around.

Once you have examined your own emotional issues, have a discussion with your partner. This may be a bit uncomfortable—especially if you aren't the type who tends to share and discuss your feelings. Establish a positive mood that allows both of you to feel comfortable vocalizing your feelings. Being open and honest will give you the best chance to enjoy a highly satisfying sexual relationship that includes BDSM.

You owe it to your partner to share your emotional triggers so that she can help you deal with them, and also so she can be prepared for any reactions or challenges you may have as you engage in your playtime activities.

Be honest about your fears, especially anything that scares you about trying specific BDSM activities. Don't worry about trying to put on a brave front. It is okay to be a bit nervous or even afraid—you are, after all, venturing into new and mysterious territory, which is bound to be a little scary. The chance to face (and hopefully overcome) your

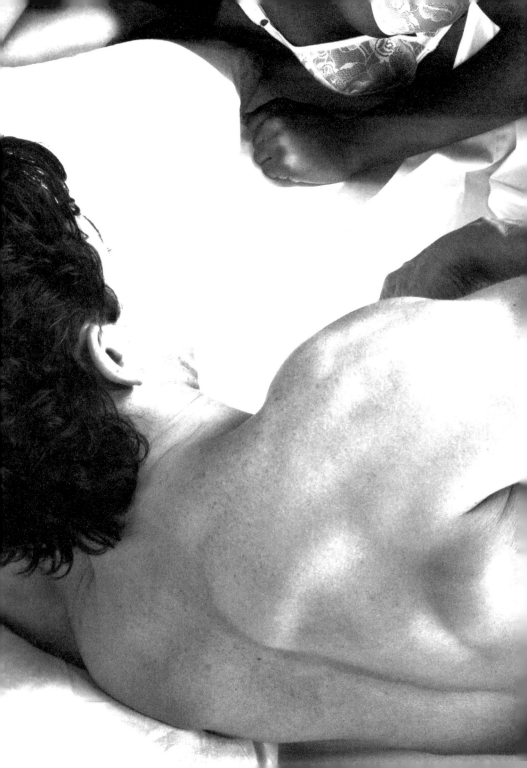

fears may add to the excitement. But you still should acknowledge and admit your fears, so that you and your partner can both tread carefully when attempting anything that might be particular frightening to you.

Obviously, this goes both ways. You must also encourage your partner to be open and honest with you—and you must do everything in your power to establish a feeling of trust that makes him feel comfortable and safe sharing his personal issues.

Even if you aren't the "touchy-feely" type and find this sort of personal sharing uncomfortable, this is an important step when embarking on a BDSM adventure. A bonus: afterwards, you will almost surely find that you and your partner have a deeper and stronger intimate bond than ever before.

Soft and Hard Limits

A big part of the process of establishing rules and boundaries is spelling out your limits. Generally, two types of limits are used in BDSM arrangements: hard limits and soft limits. In both cases, you want to take time to think about them and be sure to spell them out specifically. Don't assume your partner can read your mind and know what you are or are not comfortable with. Likewise, do not take it for granted that your partner will be really into a certain act, only to discover the hard way that she is strongly opposed to it.

Soft Limits

You might think of soft limits as the negotiable areas. These are things you are unsure about, but may be willing to try at some time. You might want to add some additional disclaimers to your soft limits. For example, you might say that you would consider anal play once you have become comfortable with other "warm-up" activities and provided you have taken steps beforehand to ensure you are fully ready. Or you might stipulate that you would consider using a spreader bar after you have tried softer restraints and felt okay with them.

Some people view soft limits as an "I'll try anything once" type of thing. This is your opportunity to experiment with areas that may seem foreign and mysterious to you, and explore your unknown turn-ons, possibly discovering a few you never knew you had. On the other hand, it is also a way to determine if you truly do not like a specific activity.

The important thing to remember is that soft limits can be revisited and renegotiated as you proceed with your BDSM explorations. If you try something once and don't like it, you can always shift it from your soft limits list to the hard limits category. And when it comes to your partner's soft limits, you need to respect her right to do the same thing.

Hard Limits

Hard limits are the nonnegotiable conditions of your agreement. These are the things you definitely will not try, and will not even consider. If you are simply unsure about something or have any thoughts that you might want to try it at some point, put it on your soft limits list for now—you can always change it later.

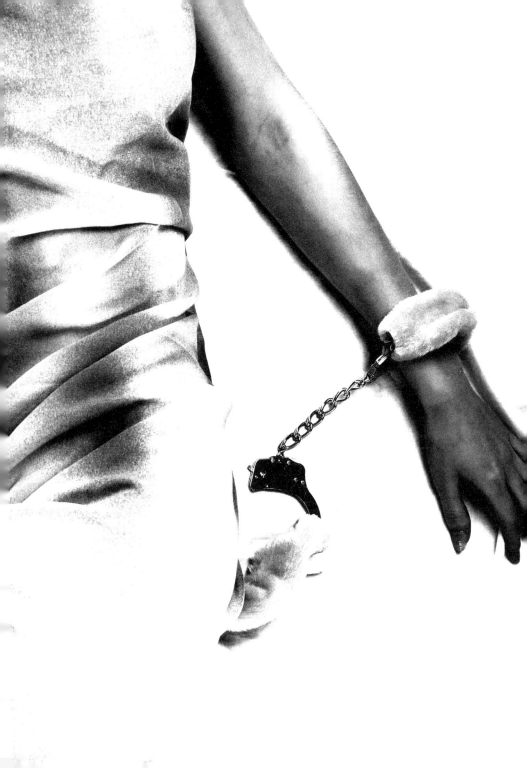

You must respect your partner's hard limits, just as you would expect your partner to respect yours. Never try to convince him to do something he has already put on his list of hard limits.

Safe Is Sexy

In addition to hard and soft limits, some contracts also provide for the submissive (or both parties) to have "veto" power under certain circumstances. This may also be given as a reward. Or the submissive may start out with a certain number of veto allowances—sort of like "get out of jail free" cards—which she may use as she wishes.

Safe Words

Any discussion of boundaries and limits with regards to BDSM will almost always include a mention of "safe words" and how to use them. Safe words are critical in letting your partner know when you want to stop or slow down the action. They work like a referee's whistle or a stop sign. Here are some tips to using BDSM safe words effectively:

- Don't rely on words such as "no" or "stop." You need specific and unique safe words because people often yell out words like "no" in the throes of passion instinctively, even though they really do not want their partners to stop what they are doing.

palomino

safe word

potato

foliage

kumquat

banana

YELLOW

green

flugelhorn Wyoming

Arnie

quail

RED

ice cream man

ziggurat

pinech

Gibson lemon

apples

pineapple

whiskey

pizza TROLLEY

- Use odd or unusual words. The more unique, the more likely they are to send a clear message, and the less likely that confusion will result.
- Consider using code words of various categories. You might want to choose some words to mean you are nearing your limits, and other words to mean you want to stop right now.
- Don't jump the gun or use these words excessively. If you frequently yell your safe words as soon as the action gets started, you will only frustrate your partner—and neither of you will have a good time. If you find yourself using safe words a lot, it may be time to reevaluate your limits and consider your comfort level regarding the activities you are trying.

To add an extra element of fun, casually find ways to drop your safe words into seemingly innocent conversations while you and your partner are out in public. This will be like a naughty inside secret between the two of you.

Contracts

The heart of every BDSM arrangement is the contract. This is the ultimate agreement, which must be respected and followed by both partners at all times. You will want to work on drafting your contract as soon as you start thinking about trying any BDSM activities. This way you'll have all your rules and guidelines in place right from the start, which will help you avoid problems later.

Contracts can be written documents or verbal agreements, whichever you and your partner prefer. Many people decide to put a contract in writing, because then it is very clear and there is less chance for confusion or for one person to forget or misunderstand the rules. Needless to say, a written contract for BDSM purposes is purely a symbolic gesture, albeit a serious and important one. It isn't likely to be considered official or binding in a court of law. Still, it should only be used by consenting adults of legal age.

If you are turned off by the formality of putting together a written contract, be creative in coming up with ways to make the process sexier. For example, you could incorporate it into a "boss and secretary" role-playing fantasy. Or you could reward yourselves with X-rated treats for each section you complete.

You can also make your contract as formal or graphic as you wish. Some couples find it entertaining and exciting to use a lot of "dirty words" in a written contract that otherwise looks very official.

As with any type of contract or agreement, the issues and interests of both parties should be addressed. You will want to cover the rights and responsibilities of the person in the submissive role as well as those of the person in the dominant role. Spell out what is expected of each person, covering every minor rule you think should be included.

You and your partner should both have an equal and active say in drafting the contract. Regardless of who will be the dominant, nobody is the boss at this stage in the relationship. Each should have the ability

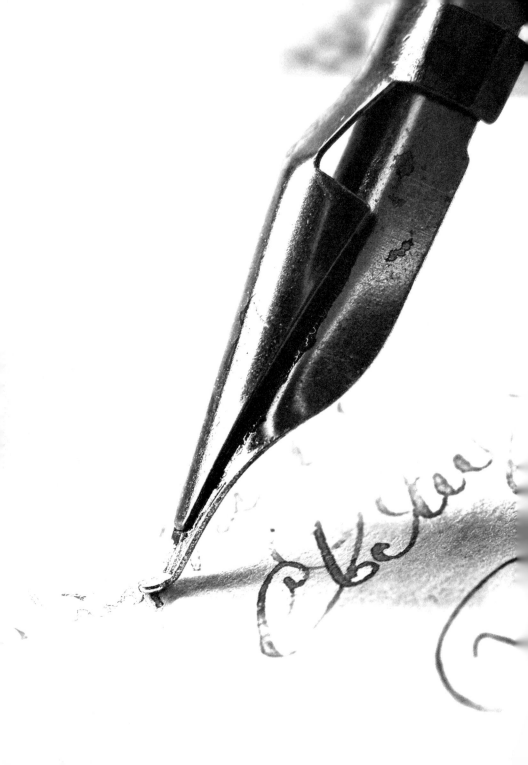

to negotiate and discuss any point of concern. Ideally, you will find a way to reach a mutually agreeable compromise in areas where you have differing opinions.

Neither partner should sign—or agree to, in the case of a verbal contract—the agreement until he or she is totally ready and feels comfortable with everything in the agreement. Take your time with this important step, and don't rush yourself or your partner to agree before both of you feel ready.

Safe Is Sexy

What should you include in your contract? Start with the basics, such as hard and soft limits and any major rules you feel are important. After that, it is up to you. You can include whatever you want. Decide what are priorities for you, but feel free to also include some whimsical and fun stuff—like what playlists you will use as background music for specific activities or the types of decorations that are off limits for your playroom.

When drafting a BDSM agreement, many people also include punishments and rewards. These consequences are incurred when one partner (generally the submissive) pleases or displeases the other. Such contracts are sometimes referred to in the BDSM community as "slave contracts" because they are used to indicate the master or dominant's (symbolic) "ownership" of a sex slave.

These items are commonly included in a dominant/submissive contract:

- Rights and responsibilities of both parties
- Hard and soft limits
- Duration of the agreement (when the contract expires, or is up for renegotiation)
- Punishments and rewards
- Details of what (if any) sexual activities or partners are allowed outside of the relationship
- Personal preferences (generally of the dominant)

A wide variety of sample BDSM contracts are available online. Use a search engine to find some examples or browse large BDSM community websites.

Chapter 4

Playing with Toys

> *"I can remember when the air
> was clean and sex was dirty."*
>
> —George Burns

A dominant is often only as good as the toys in his arsenal. An impressive and fully stocked treasure chest is worth its weight in gold. BDSM is all about play, after all—so the more toys you have, the more fun the experience will be for you and your partner.

To add to the excitement and anticipation, keep your treasure chest locked or make it off-limits to your partner. That way, you can reveal your toys one at a time as you are ready to work them into your sex play. You will keep your partner on his toes with your endless series of sexy surprises! And if you catch your partner snooping, you can always punish him with some spankings.

 Kinky Tip

Let you partner create a "wish list" of toys and accessories she would like to try. It is then up to you to decide whether to include those items on your shopping list. You may use them as rewards if your partner pleases you. Ideally, you should try to put a creative spin on the requested items or add some sort of fun "extra," just to give things an unexpected twist. For example, if your partner mentions a curiosity about handcuffs, maybe you can find some furry handcuffs in her favorite color, or a shade that happens to match a scarf or necktie you have—so they can be used together as a set.

What should you include in your toy box, treasure chest, or playroom supply closet? That's a matter of personal preference, and will often depend on the specific activities you plan to engage in with your partner. Discovering your own special and unique toys is half the fun.

But some basic "sex supply staples" are considered standard for most playrooms.

Feathers, Scarves, and Other Tame Toys

Probably the easiest (and least intimidating) toys to start with are the innocent looking and readily available things like scarves and feathers. One advantage of these types of toys is that you can easily find them anywhere. You can also buy them at your local store without any embarrassment. If you or your partner is a bit timid or nervous about purchasing or playing with toys, this can be a relatively tame way to take that first step.

But just because scarves aren't necessarily as shocking or risqué as some other toys in your arsenal doesn't mean they can't be sexy or exciting. There are lots of ways to up the ante and add an extra element of spice to these common items. For example, you could spray the scarves with your favorite perfume or cologne—or better yet, find a creative way to infuse them with your own intimate body scents.

The same goes for feathers. You can use feathers and scarves to create a special sexy outfit for yourself or your partner—which can then be modeled and incorporated into your sensual bedroom routine, and removed in passion later.

When using toys at the mild end of the spectrum, add creativity and imagination. Conjure up an X-rated scenario or role-playing adventure using scarves and/or feathers. Or use them to tease your

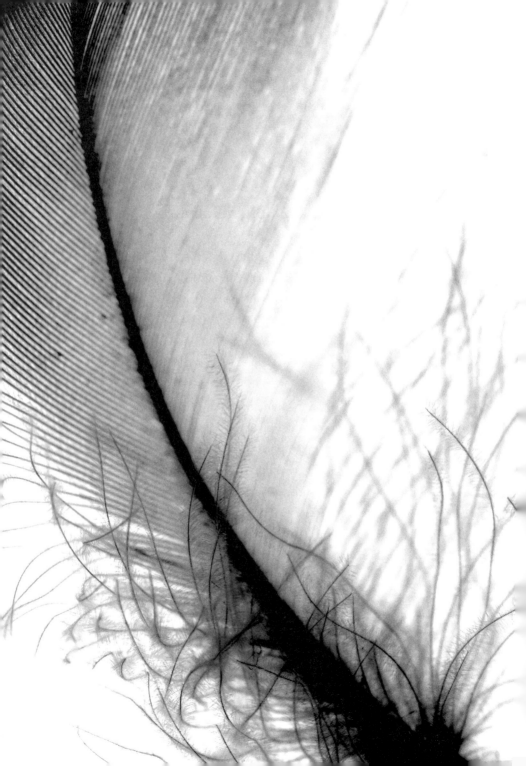

partner, exquisitely torturing her by slowly running the feather lightly along her thighs or breasts. Tickle her in sensitive areas. Tantalize her by dancing the feathers over her erogenous zones. Using this to build anticipation will help you get to the point where your lover is begging you to take things further.

Kinky Tip

You can incorporate a feather duster into a "sex slave" or role-playing game. Order your submissive to dress up in a sexy servant outfit—or perhaps as a nude housecleaner—and have him do some household chores with the same feather duster you will use to tease him later. This will allow your lover to imagine the sweet torture you have planned after his chores are done.

To get the maximum benefit, combine feather teasing with licking, nibbling, and other moves that will get your partner hot and have her squirming in pleasure. Many people enjoy combining feathers with blindfolds. If your partner cannot see, she will be hypersensitive to even the lightest touch, and your feather teasing will feel even more amazing.

Scarves are other seemingly innocent toys that can be used in all sorts of creative and naughty ways. Like neckties, scarves can become restraints when you first start out in BDSM activities. (See Chapter 7 for more information and suggestions for using different types of restraints.)

Again, you can work scarves into your role-playing games or other warm-up activities. Use them to create a gypsy costume for your submissive, and then order her to remove it as part of a sexy striptease for you. You can also put some extra intimate meaning into your choice of scarves. Maybe you can devise a "color code" in which certain shades act as a signal for what you have planned for your partner. A red scarf, for example, silently announces to your submissive that he will be spanked at some time in the evening.

To encourage unique physical sensations, try creating (or order your submissive to create) scarves from different types of material—some soft, some rough. You can even go on a sexy shopping spree together to a craft store to pick out material to turn into homemade scarves.

Tip: a feather boa can do double duty, providing the soft teasing benefits of feathers as well as serving as a makeshift scarf for restraint activities. And, of course, it is a great accoutrement for a sexy striptease.

Vibrators

Vibrators may be common, but that does not mean they are boring. Vibrators come in all sorts of styles, colors, materials, and models, from basic, no-frills types to fancy, high-tech kinds with lots of varying speeds and settings that do just about everything but take out the trash.

Incorporating vibrators into your sex play offers numerous advantages. For one thing, it is likely that your partner has some experience with them or at least is familiar with how they work. If your partner has little or no experience in this area, you can start with one of the basic models just to get her comfortable with the concept—most likely, she will quickly become a fan and eagerly invite you to take things up a notch by adding some more advanced models to your toy chest.

Another tip for newbies: start with a low speed setting and gradually adjust it as you find your comfort level. A high speed can often be too intense for those who aren't prepared for or familiar with the sensation.

Another upside of vibrators is that, to put it simply, they get the job done. They're very efficient and effective at getting your partner revved up in a short period of time. Positioning the vibrator on a woman's sweet spot (being careful to approach it gradually and keep the pressure at just the right level) can bring her close to the point of climax quickly.

Vibrators can also be a great way to tease your partner. Many models allow you to control them from a distance, so you can stop and start the vibration as you wish. This is a great way to bring your partner to the brink repeatedly—or if you feel like punishing her, getting her frustrated.

Some types of vibrating toys, such as vibrating panties, allow you to use a remote control and take your partner by complete surprise when she least expects it. You can even order your submissive to wear vibrating panties underneath her clothes while you are out in public— you can then watch her squirm as you enjoy playing with the remote control.

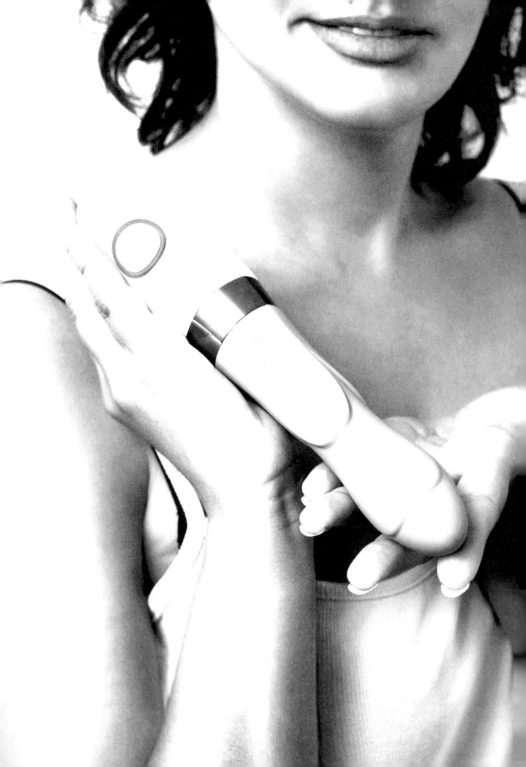

Half the fun of using vibrators is experimenting with lots of different models and features. No matter what you are into, you'll probably find several different vibrators that will meet your needs. One popular variety is the "two-headed" style, which stimulates two areas at once, say, the clitoris and vagina, or the vagina and the anus. A few triple-headed models are also available, for the ultimate in stimulating pleasure!

Many vibrators are designed with a cock-like appearance, allowing them to give you the look and feel of a dildo when inserted. For the ultimate sensual torture, tease your partner by inserting it very slowly while also adjusting the speeds. Other styles feature beads or balls on the part designed for insertion, which adds thrilling sensations.

Safe Is Sexy

If you are going to bring a vibrator into the shower or bathtub, choose a model that is specifically designed to be used in water—many waterproof varieties are available.

Although more commonly used on and by women, vibrators are increasingly used to pleasure men, as well. Hold a vibrator against the man's sensitive areas, experimenting to find the position and approach that drives him wild. Vibrating cock rings work well, too. Some vibrators are designed for couples to use together, and feature a cock ring attached to the phallic-shaped vibrator. Anal vibrators can be enjoyed by partners of either gender. (See the section on anal toys later in this chapter for more information.)

Dildos

Dildos have become viewed as an old-school sex toy, now that vibrators have stolen their thunder. But don't count the dildo out just yet—it can still be a very exciting toy, in the right hands.

Like the vibrator the dildo comes in lots of different styles. Part of the allure of the dildo is it provides the physical sensation and the visual image of insertion, which can be exciting to the person experiencing it as well as the person watching the action. Many men find this to be a huge turn-on, as it can be like watching their partners have sex with other men—especially now that many dildos have a very lifelike appearance.

Safe Is Sexy

With dildos and vibrators (and probably most sex toys in general), you often get what you pay for. Many adult toy websites abound with negative reviews from customers who are disappointed with the cheaper products, which often have unappealing aspects such as a bad smell or the tendency to fall apart easily. This is definitely one case where it pays to splurge. You and your partner are worth it!

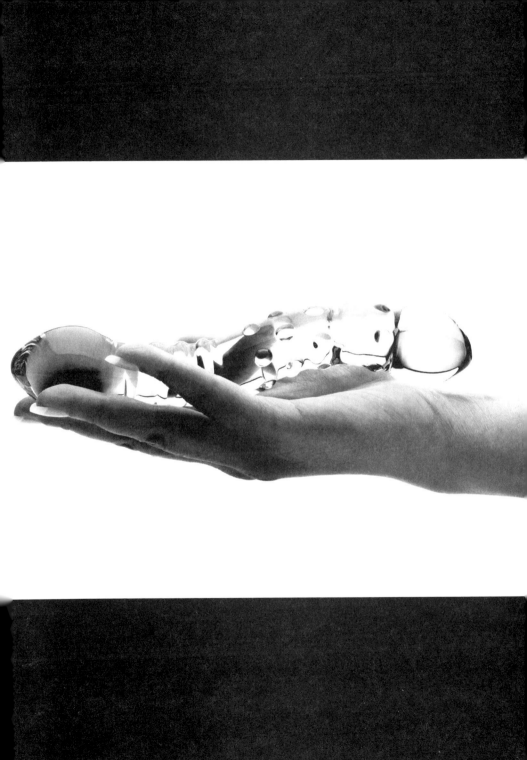

Dildos are not just for use on women. Women can use "strap-ons" with either their male or female partners. Couples can use a two-ended dildo—sometimes referred to as "double dongs"—together. (These can be used either by lesbian couples who both want vaginal penetration at the same time, or by heterosexual couples—the man would be penetrated anally while the woman is penetrated either anally or vaginally.) Dildos specifically designed for anal use can be enjoyed by couples of any sexual persuasion.

Tip: if you or your partner is inexperienced with condoms and the correct way to put them on, a dildo can be a great tool to help you practice your technique.

Here are some tips for selecting and using a dildo:

- If you are new to this type of toy, begin with a smaller size. Not only does it look less intimidating, it will be easier for you to insert.
- If you are aiming for maximum arousal visually, look for one that appears as lifelike as possible.
- Make sure to use lots of lube, and begin by inserting slowly, especially if the dildo is on the larger side.
- Keep dildos (and all sex toys) clean. Wash with mild soap and water after each use. Some people also use a condom on the dildo, to reduce the risk of germs or bacteria remaining on the toy.

Dildos and vibrators designed for insertion are made from several different materials. Rubber or jelly-type materials allow for greater flexibility. Others are made from a more solid substance, which provides a firmer feel that some people prefer. Many people have a preference for one type or another, so you may want to experiment with different styles to determine which you like best.

Ben Wa Balls

Many people are unfamiliar with Ben Wa Balls—but that just makes them a more exciting addition to your treasure chest. Your partner probably hasn't used them before (especially if she is relatively inexperienced or new to the BDSM lifestyle) so this will give you the chance to surprise her with something totally new and enticing.

Said to be one of the oldest sex toys designed for women's pleasure, Ben Wa Balls are usually believed to have originated in Asian cultures (some legends say they were used by geishas to perfect their sexual skills and strengthen their pelvic muscles). Ben Wa Balls are sometimes referred to by other names, including "orgasm balls" and "Venus balls." They are inserted in the vagina and can be kept there for a period of time to heighten arousal and to serve as a teaser. They are available in different sizes and can be made from a variety of materials, including soft jelly/rubber substances, metal, or glass. Some styles even vibrate and can be operated with a remote control. The balls are generally configured in a row of two or more, attached together in a chain formation with an extra length of material at the end to allow them to be extracted from the body easily.

Traditional Ben Wa Balls were commonly sold as separate, unconnected balls, without any sort of "chain" attached. However, those types

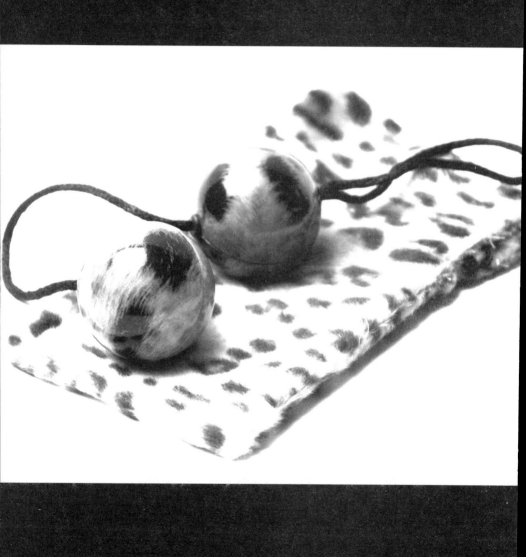

of balls have become less popular with many people who fear the balls can get "lost" inside a woman—plus, they can be a little more challenging to remove. Women who are experienced with using applicator-less tampons and similar inserted products are more likely to be comfortable using loose Ben Wa Balls. Bonus: these balls can also be a great way to exercise your Kegel muscles.

Ben Wa Balls can be a bit of a shock at first, but can provide a uniquely erotic sensation—especially if you insert them and leave them in while you move around. You can order your partner to keep them in for a period of time—say, as the two of you attend a public event—to really extend the sensation and heighten the excitement.

Again, the rule of thumb is to start small and slow. At first, choose balls that are on the smaller side—say, the size of a small stone—until you get comfortable with the idea of having them inside of you. You may want to add some lube, if the balls are made from a lube-friendly material. (As a general rule, items made from silicone or latex should only be used with water-based lubricants, and metal objects may not be designed for use with lube, so read the directions or packaging.) It is also fun to experiment with exactly how you position the balls for maximum pleasure. This varies from one person to another; some like them inserted more deeply, others prefer to have them just barely inside, so they can stimulate the sensitive nerve endings.

You can build anticipation by first putting the balls in your mouth or your partner's, after announcing that the balls will soon be slipped inside your partner. Bonus: this adds a little extra lubrication to the balls.

A big part of the erotic thrill of using Ben Wa Balls is removing them. They can be removed by pulling on the string-like portion at the end, either slowly or quickly as your mood suggests. One technique is to pull them out quickly just before or in conjunction with the woman's climax, to supercharge her orgasm. Ben Wa Balls can also be used for anal pleasure by people of either sex. Experiment with different approaches to find the one you enjoy most—or the one that allows you to best tease your partner.

Anal Toys

If you enjoy anal stimulation—or are unsure if you do and want to slowly explore that type of activity—anal toys can be a great addition to your toy chest. You'll find several varieties from which to choose. These can often be a good way to "warm up" to the idea of anal play if you are not quite ready to try anal sex, as in, penetration with your partner's finger or penis.

The most common types of anal toys are beads and plugs. Anal beads are somewhat similar to Ben Wa Balls, although they are generally smaller. They are arranged in a strand or chain formation, usually consisting of several beads, possibly as many as ten. Often, the beads gradually increase in size as the strand progresses—which adds an extra exciting sensation and can also be a good way to help you slowly adjust to different sizes.

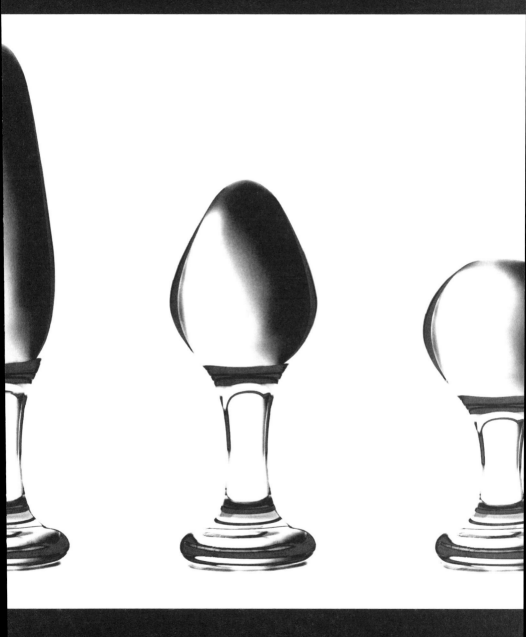

As with Ben Wa Balls, it is important to proceed slowly. Insert one bead at a time and give yourself time in between to adapt to the sensation.

Anal beads come in vibrating styles—the vibration combined with the slow and gradual insertion of the strand of beads can really drive you or your partner wild! Although many straight men are initially skittish about any sort of anal insertion, vibrating anal beads can be a special thrill for them if they give it a chance—the sensation of having a vibrating object inside of them is more of a rare treat for men than for women.

Anal plugs (also commonly known as butt plugs) are similar to dildos, although generally much smaller. Like dildos, they come in a variety of styles and substances. They are often used to "train" the anal area and get it (and the person) warmed up for the initial foray into anal sex.

Like anal beads, anal plugs are available in vibrating styles—which again can be very arousing for a man. These plugs are said to be an effective way to stimulate the prostate for a powerful orgasm experience.

Again, it is important to follow the cardinal rules: Start slowly, proceed at your own pace, and use plenty of lube.

Chapter 5

A Place to Play

"Women need a reason to have sex. Men just need a place."

—Billy Crystal

Realtors say the most important thing about a property is "location, loca-tion, location." Well, this can be an important element in sex play, as well. When it comes to getting your partner or yourself in the mood for some steamy action, location matters. Choosing the right setting and creating a sexy environment can go a long way toward establishing the right mood.

Even if you are already well on your way to being turned on, the right setting can really help enhance your passionate mood. On the other hand, the wrong setting can kill your buzz as fast as a cold shower. Who wants to engage in some hot and heavy action in a messy, depressing, or just plain bland environment? Granted, if you are excited enough, you can ignore the setting—and in some cases a cold or sterile setting may even work to your advantage, say, if you are doing some sort of role-playing game, or if you want to make things cold or uncomfortable for your submissive.

But most of the time—especially if you are trying something new or are a little bit nervous or apprehensive and may be slow to get warmed up—the setting can play a big part in making or breaking your sexual action.

Think of yourself as a star getting ready for your big performance. You may be motivated and excited about giving an amazing perfor-mance, but you still need the scenery and props to help you get into character and establish the right mood.

If you want to surprise your partner and perhaps make it easier to seduce him or her, choosing or creating the right setting can give you a big head start in getting both of you in the mood. And if you are the dominant, your partner may expect you to create the setting as part of your arrangement.

Don't underestimate the importance of this job. Think about some of your most exciting sexual encounters. What do you remember most about the experience? Yes, the partner and positions are probably memorable—but chances are good you remember stuff related to the setting, like the feeling of the soft furniture and bedding, the smell of the candles, the sounds of romantic or sexy music, and more. Remember, this is a "sensual" experience. All your senses are involved—and tend to be hypersensitive when you are excited. You want to make this a supremely intoxicating experience for all your partner's senses—which will make it even more unforgettable for both of you.

The Bedroom

For many people, the bedroom is the most obvious sexual setting. It is the most common—and often the most easily accessible—place for us to enjoy some alone time with our partners. But the fact that it is so obvious and normal can be both a blessing and a curse. On the one hand, it will likely feel comfortable and familiar. This is especially helpful when you are trying new activities that might be a bit intimidating. Having a comfortable place where you feel relaxed and at ease can be a big advantage in this case.

On the other hand, many of us have a tendency to become a little (or a lot) too comfortable in our bedrooms. Frankly, many bedrooms today are far from sexy or romantic. They may contain desks, electronics, and other work supplies. Our bedrooms often resemble

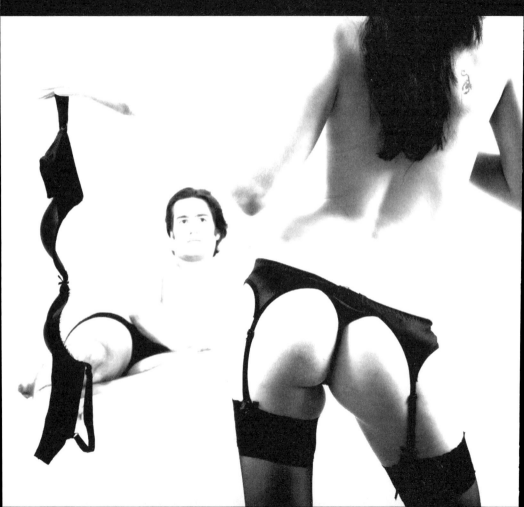

mini-offices. And who wants to have hot steamy action in the same place where you have conference calls with the office?

When evaluating why some couples have a lack, or at least a slow-down, of action in the bedroom, the bedroom itself can hold a lot of clues. Many relationship experts (and passionate couples) strongly believe that the bedroom should be solely for sleeping and sex. Filling it with lots of other clutter—and uses—makes it less special and can often make you view your bedroom as a place you don't enjoy, as opposed to someplace where you can escape and have fun.

Your bedroom should be a private oasis, where you can relax, recharge, and revel in some thrilling alone time with your significant other. It should be your love nest—or to put it a bit more adult, your spicy sensual playground.

If you want to spice up your bedroom action, spend some time evaluating and improving the room, from a sexiness standpoint. Make this your pleasure palace—or at least a sexy retreat. Start with the bed and transform it into a sensual paradise. Invest in some satin sheets in black, red, or an animal print. Get rid of kids' toys, clutter, and anything work-related. Set up some romantic lighting.

Remember to pay attention to scents and sounds, too. Many people underestimate the importance of these elements—but all your senses will be heightened when you are aroused (especially if you will be restrained or blindfolded). Lots of studies show that scents trigger chemical responses in our brains. Certain scents, such as patchouli, musk, ylang-ylang, and jasmine, are said to have aphrodisiac qualities—although each of us has unique, individual preferences. Do some experimenting to find the ones that work their magic on you and your partner.

You will, of course, want to add some extra elements to make your bedroom more BDSM-friendly. This will depend on exactly what activities you plan to try, and how private your bedroom really is. If it is strictly a place for the two of you, you don't need to be so covert. However, if other people (such as children, or even a house-keeper) occasionally come into your bedroom, you probably don't want to have a big X-cross attached to the wall or a suspension grid affixed to the ceiling. But you can keep some scarves next to the bed, and perhaps stash a pair of cuffs and a paddle or other spanking toys underneath it.

You may be able to keep all your toys in your bedroom closet or dresser drawer. But it will be more exciting if you invest in a special "treasure chest" where you can store your sex supplies.

Kinky Tip

If your partner doesn't live in the same place as you, or will be away for at least a few days, surprise him or her with a sexy bedroom makeover. Be creative and put emphasis on making the room sex-friendly—in other words, passionate and playful. If your bedroom has gotten too comfortable and has a "lived in" look, a radical change can be just the spark you need to supercharge your sex life. As an extra special touch, try to work in things that are part of a special theme or have inside meaning for both of you. For example, if you will be ordering your submissive partner to dress up like a maid, a few feather dusters used as decorative accessories can send her a little signal of what you have planned.

When setting up the bedroom for maximum sexual pleasure, don't forget the mirror(s). You probably have at least one somewhere in the bedroom already, but selecting one that's the perfect size (a full-length one is a great choice) and positioning it in just the right spot can help you both enjoy some thrilling visual images while sexually pleasuring yourselves and each other.

If you and your partner aren't able to get away from home as much as you would like, try adding a few touches that make the bedroom feel like a resort or hotel. Perhaps you can design your own special "Do Not Disturb" sign while you are at it!

Living Room

When selecting a room in the house for sex play, the living room is perhaps the second-best (or the second most common) choice. This is mainly because—like the bedroom—it tends to have soft furniture that is conducive to lying or sitting on, and that allows you to get into all sorts of positions and arrangements. The living room can also seem a little more exciting than the bedroom, because sex play here it isn't quite so routine.

The living room can have some pros and cons as a sex setting. As just mentioned, it is already stocked with some important supplies —furniture and possibly pillows or throws. And, as with the bed-room, is probably feels cozy and familiar to you, which can help you feel relaxed. The fact that it is not as private as the bedroom can add an exciting element of danger or naughtiness to your living room encounters—you could be "caught in the act" if someone pops over for an unannounced visit.

Often, living rooms have supplies that can come in handy for ramping up the sexual excitement. The television, for instance. If you have cable channels, it's likely that you can find some adult entertainment on at least a few channels. Or, you can surprise your partner with a special DVD that features his or her turn-ons. A stereo or CD player with your own "passion playlist" can also help establish the right mood.

If you and your partner have gotten into a "bedroom only" pattern, take advantage of the novelty of getting intimate in the living room. Maybe you can work this new location into a fantasy or role-playing game. Pretend you and your partner are teenagers who are supposed to be studying or watching television in the living room—but of course you naughty kids decide to enjoy a covert make-out session (and more) while trying not to wake up anyone else in the house and hoping your parents don't catch you.

Don't overlook the props you can find in the living room that might lend themselves well to some BDSM play. Scarves or curtain ties can serve as good bondage supplies. A footstool or ottoman can be a great place for the submissive to get into position for a spanking.

Although the living room definitely has passionate potential, it can also have a few downsides. The "public" nature of the living room, though exciting in some ways, can be a drawback. If there are other people living in the house, the living room may not offer you the privacy you want. It may even be tough to find a time when you can be alone in that room.

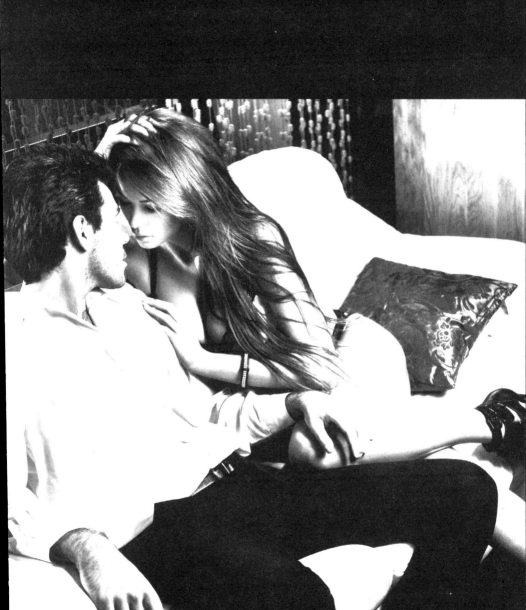

Even if you don't live with anyone else, the living room may still be a bit too visible or accessible for your comfort. If it is connected to or near the front door you run the risk of being interrupted by a deliveryman (or worse, a relative who decides to drop in for a surprise visit), though some people may find that possibility a turn-on. In most houses, the living room is on the first floor so people passing by might be able to see in through the windows. Again, this may be a turn-on or a turn-off for you.

And, as with the bedroom, the living room may be a little too "lived in" to really let you feel sexy. It can be tough to muster up your inner sex goddess if you are surrounded by video games, schoolbooks, or other everyday household items.

But if you decide to "christen" the living room as one of your play locations, give it a few sexy elements. You will probably need to be more subtle or discreet than with your bedroom décor, but try to find a few ways to add some sexy accessories that will have private meaning for your and your partner. For example, you could tie the curtains with a sash that you also use for bondage play.

Kitchen

The kitchen can be a surprisingly common setting for sex—or at least for some hot and steamy foreplay. You can probably think of a few memorable scenes from movies or television in which couples frantically went at it on a kitchen table or counter (think *Fatal Attraction* or *The Postman Always Rings Twice*).

The kitchen probably does not have the comfy furniture you might find in your bedroom or living room. Most kitchens are full of hard and cold surfaces. But that can be exactly what makes this such an exciting environment for sex—especially the kind of frantic, "rip your clothes off in urgent passion" action you see in the movies. The kitchen feels sterile and practical, which can make it seem like you are breaking the rules by doing something sexual and personal there.

From a logistical standpoint, the kitchen offers new and unique possibilities for creative positions. Most likely, at least one of you will need to be on a counter or table. The cold and hard surfaces will also present some new sensations for your skin, making this a novel and thrilling experience.

You can even take a cue from Hollywood and reenact some classic kitchen-sex moves, such as clearing off the table in one big sweep. (The submissive partner may have to clean up the mess later.) It's a good idea to remove any glass jars or breakable items first, to avoid the risk of accidental injury.

As a bonus, the kitchen is stocked with items that can come in very handy for sex in general, but especially for more risqué play like BDSM. You will have easy access to things like spatulas, wooden spoons, and other utensils that can serve as great makeshift paddles. Potholders, hand towels, and other kitchen linens can also be worked into your play in all sorts of creative ways—such as using them as makeshift blindfolds or just for padding when you will be lying on or against hard kitchen surfaces.

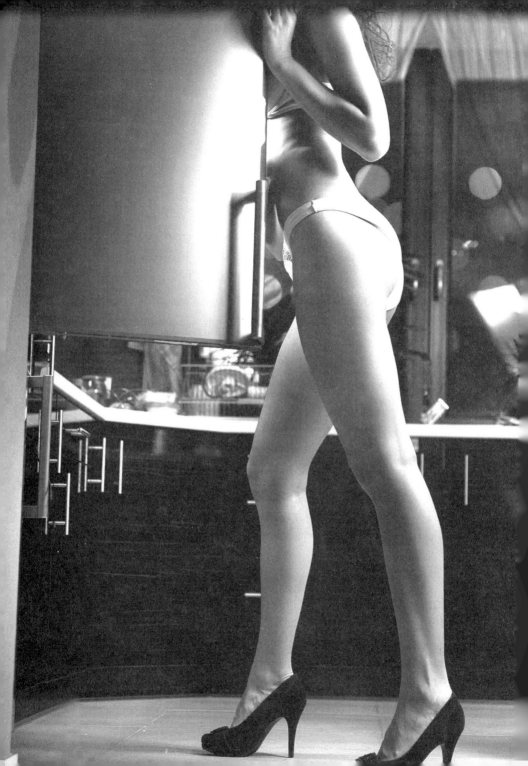

Then, of course, there are all sorts of food-related options. You can help yourself to chocolate sauce, whipped cream, cherries, and other treats from the fridge. Again, be creative—don't forget the fruit and vegetable drawers. Ice cubes and other frozen treats can also act as stimulating sex toys.

Yes, you may make quite a mess—but you can always hose each other down or soap each other up in the sink. (If that's not possible or you need to get a little cleaner, you can always head to the bathroom for some soapy shower action.)

Again, a downside of the kitchen is that it tends to be one of the most visible and public areas of the house. If you don't live alone, the risk of getting caught or interrupted may be either a turn-on or a deterrent, depending on your viewpoint. Not to mention, the other members of the household may not be overjoyed to learn what you've been doing on the table where they eat their morning oatmeal.

On the plus side, the kitchen offers lots of sexy role-playing opportunities. You can pretend to be the bored housewife and the appliance repairman, or even just a seemingly boring married couple (think *Leave It to Beaver*) who are suddenly so overtaken with passion that they must have each other right there on the kitchen counter.

Even when the actual sex itself does not take place in the kitchen, this room can still play a role in your sex life. Many couples spend a lot of time in the kitchen—eating, preparing meals, or just having conversations. This can be important quality time that can help your relationship. It can also serve as good foreplay. You can enjoy some playful touching and flirting while preparing dinner—and don't miss the opportunity to feed each other bites of food in sensuous ways. You can also make a routine of talking dirty at the dinner table (provided it is just the two of you) as a warm-up for the action later in the bedroom. This sexual tension can be very titillating—and can really make you start to look forward to mealtime in a whole new way!

Game Room, Office, or Library

Once you have explored (or ruled out) the bedroom, living room, and kitchen as good sex spots, think about other rooms in your home that might offer a more creative and unusual option. If you have a large home, there could be lots of possibilities. But even a smaller place may offer at least one not-so-obvious sex hideaway. Even a decent-sized closet could do in a pinch.

A game room is a perfect choice. Climb on top of, or lean against, a pool, ping pong, or poker table. Recliners, sofas, or other furniture will also come in handy. Look around for "toys" that can be used in adult ways, for example, billiard balls, ping pong paddles, or cue sticks.

A home office can also be a great choice because it offers the best of both worlds. It affords the furniture and horizontal surfaces that come in handy, but also has a more formal, businesslike feeling that can be an exciting novelty. The "naughty" idea that you are breaking the rules by having such erotic pleasure in a place that is presumably meant for serious business can be enticing. And, of course, it is the perfect place for role-playing scenarios involving the boss and secretary.

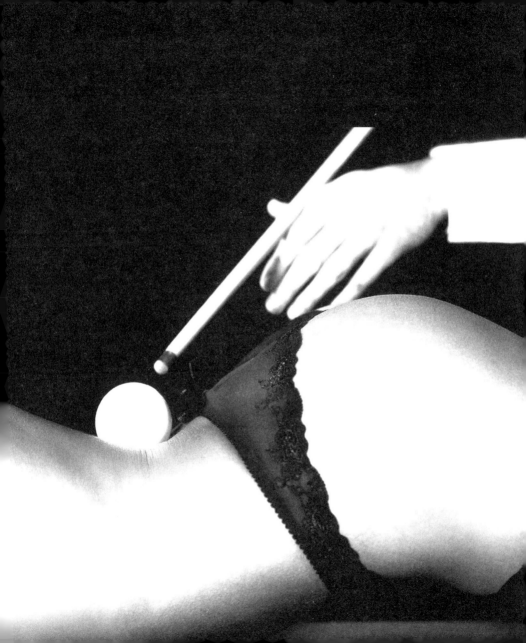

Many offices and dens also tend to have a somewhat masculine feel, which can make them the perfect antidote to the bedroom, which often has a more feminine feel. If the man is the dominant, this can help establish his role as the one with the power in this environment, and can reinforce the idea that this is his domain.

If you happen to have a library in your home, or even just an area with some bookshelves and a desk, don't pass up the opportunity to do a "naughty librarian" or "sexy teacher" scenario. Be sure to stock the shelves with some X-rated literature you can read to each other to get in the mood. You can even hide a few treats or toys behind the books as a surprise.

Kinky Tip

Make it your sexual mission to "christen" each room in the house, except perhaps bedrooms that don't belong to either of you. Devise creative strategies or scenarios for getting it on in some of the more public areas of the house. To make it even more fun, you might want to create a map of your home and mark specific destinations for your sexy tour—perhaps with a "treasure" hidden at a special location. Put a gold star on each room on the map once you have "conquered" it. Need inspiration? While watching porn, make it a point to look for non-bedroom sex scenes and then try to reenact them in various rooms in your own house.

The Bathroom

You have probably already included the bathroom in your sex play, at least in some manner, but how you utilize it may depend upon its size and setup. If you are lucky enough to have a whirlpool bathtub, it's a no-brainer to take advantage of that location for some slippery fun in the hot bubbles. Naturally, you'll want to make good use of those pulsing water jets, too.

Virtually every bathroom has a shower, where you can wash each other's bodies in all those deliciously "dirty" spots and enjoy the lubrication of the hot, soapy water. This is also a great place to engage in sex while standing up. Be sure any sex toys or other supplies you use here are waterproof and safe for use when wet. You may also want to look into toys designed specifically for bathroom use, such as dildos with suction cup attachments that can be affixed to the floor or a tub or shower.

If your bathroom only has a tiny tub that isn't big enough for two people, you can still work it into your foreplay. If only one of you can fit in it, the other can stand nearby and wash or massage the bathing person. The submissive can be blindfolded while the dominant scrubs her, or he can order her to clean herself according to his specifications. And don't rule out a powder room as a playtime possibility. We've all seen television or movie scenes of people getting it on while leaning against the bathroom sink.

The bathroom contains lots of lotions, creamy body washes, scented soaps, and other sensual delights. Be sure to take full advantage of all the options, adding lots of scent-sational variety.

Bonus: the bathroom almost always contains a mirror, which can add an exciting element to your sex play.

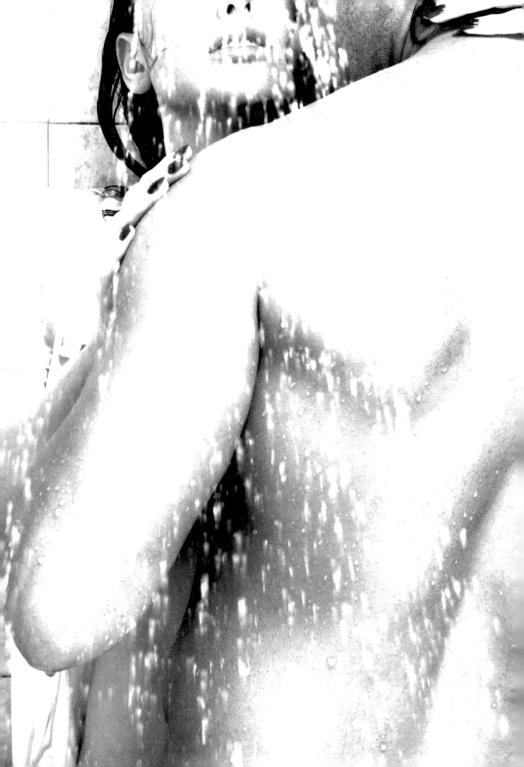

You can also incorporate some playful fun, such as snapping each other with wet towels. And the toilet (with the lid down) provides a good makeshift seating area.

Creating Your Own Playroom

If you are really serious about enjoying your BDSM activities, or just want to be able to "escape" into a special place where you can leave the real world outside, the ideal scenario is to create your own playroom, if at all possible. Obviously, this may not be an option if you have limited space—but don't automatically rule it out without at least considering your options. Do you have a guest room? A bedroom that was used by kids or other family members who have since moved out? Do you have an office or den that you don't use very often?

If you have a finished attic or basement, that could also be an option. Depending on the type of activities you will be engaging in and exactly what type of BDSM style you choose, an unfinished or semi-finished area may also be okay, and may, in fact, help set the feeling you want to create. For example, a "dungeon" type area complete with suspension cross or restraints may be compatible with cinder block walls and other basic, primitive surroundings.

Creating a new playroom from scratch allows you to customize it exactly the way you want, with your tastes and preferences, and your partner's, in mind. You could also do this secretly, and surprise your partner with the big reveal once the playroom is completed.

A separate playroom can offer many advantages. First, this will obviously be a room just for adult play. Having a specific room dedicated solely for this purpose allows you to design it to fulfill your sexual needs perfectly. You have total freedom to be the sexpert interior decorator!

It also eliminates distractions and unsexy elements that can be a turnoff, such as work-related items or kids' toys. Every single item—furniture, decorative elements, toys, scents, sounds, etc.—in this room can be carefully chosen with your pleasure (or pain) in mind. You have the opportunity to go all out and create the ultimate playroom, limited only by your imagination (and perhaps your budget). This is your chance to make your fantasies come to life, right in your very own home.

You can also ensure total privacy by keeping this room off-limits to others. You may need to keep it locked to keep others out. If you get a lot of company or have nosy relatives, be prepared for curiosity and questions about this "secret room." You may need to come up with a cover story if you don't want people to know the truth.

Kinky Tip

What should you put in the new playroom you are creating? That's totally up to you. That's one of the best parts. This is a completely private decision based on your individual tastes and turn-ons. Most playrooms contain some standard elements—a treasure chest of toys, for example, or some sort of restraint supplies. You add the specific details. The sky is the limit, so be creative and design it to embrace and encourage all of your secret desires.

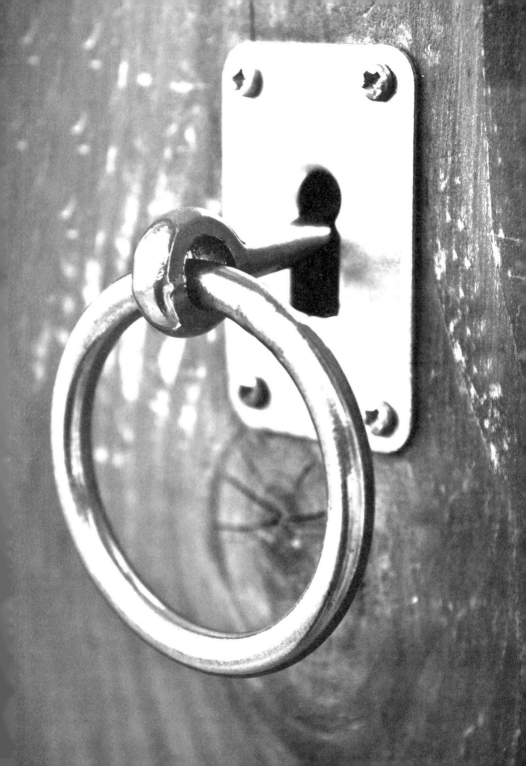

One big advantage of having a dedicated playroom is that it clearly establishes this as a place where your BDSM roles and rules are in effect. By coming through the door you shed your outside roles and instantly become Dom and Sub, or whatever titles you assign yourselves. This can be especially helpful in creating the symbolic line of separation, which defines your dominant/submissive roles as strictly for sex—they don't carry over into your everyday life. By entering the playroom, you will mentally transition to those BDSM roles.

Just knowing you have a "sex room" can be a mental turn-on. This is a luxury most people don't have, and it makes you feel special and privileged. It also makes you feel like a wild, exotic, sexual creature who isn't limited by everyday conventions. After all, boring people who have ho-hum sex lives don't have X-rated sex rooms with all sorts of shocking toys and equipment, right? Even if you didn't already feel confident and fearless at the thought of starting (or stepping up) a BDSM arrangement, this room is bound to bring out your wilder side.

Some Final Thoughts

You will probably find that having a "hot spot" that you have created (or designated) specifically for steamy sex will improve your relationship, and not just in a physical way. This "secret love nest" can strengthen your intimate bond and encourage you to spend more quality time alone together focusing solely on pleasure. It also shows that you have made your relationship a priority, which can be important for you as a couple.

Just the fact that this special space exists will make you want to make good use of it. You wouldn't want all that work you put into it to go to waste now, would you? This may give you added motivation to put some energy into creating some memorable moments in this special playroom of yours.

Even if you don't have a huge empty room at your disposal, do whatever you can to create a "sensual space" somewhere in your home. It's okay to start small, if you have to. Just get something in place while you make plans for something bigger and better.

Bonus: during a tough day at work, the mental image of what you and your partner will do to each other in your playroom that night will give you something to look forward to, and will help the day go faster—although you might find yourself squirming in your seat at the boring staff meeting.

Chapter 6

"Sense"ual Pleasure

"Sex is a part of nature.
I go along with nature."

— Marilyn Monroe

The ultimate physical experience involves all your senses. This is especially true for sexual encounters. It is called a "sensual" experience because all your senses are involved, usually to a heightened degree, when you are excited and your body is eager with anticipation. Having a fun sexual encounter is good—but having one that pleases all your senses and sends your system into overdrive is something you won't forget.

Our memories are shaped and influenced by our senses, all of them. Recall one of your most exciting moments, picturing it as clearly as you can. Most likely, you will recall not only sights, but sounds, smells, the way things felt, and possibly tasted.

Your senses can also trigger certain instinctive and automatic reactions—and, often, memories you had completely forgotten about until this moment. You have probably had an experience in which a certain smell catches you off guard and jolts you back to an important event or period in your past. Perhaps it was the certain brand of soda you always drank while at the movies with your first boyfriend. Or the perfume your hot teacher used to wear—the one that would always give you a rush when she walked a bit too close to you.

That can give you an idea of just how powerful your senses—and the experiences you associate with them—can be. They can set off a potent, almost uncontrollable reaction that can lead you to new heights of pleasure and amplify your ecstasy to unbelievable levels, sending a rush through your entire being.

You want to give yourself and your partner that type of mind-blowing, system-jolting event every time you have sex—or at least, as often as you can. It may take some effort and preparation, but anything worthwhile is worth the effort. You want to show that this is special and important. You and your partner deserve it.

The great thing is, this is easier than you might think. Yes, it does take a little preparation but it does not necessarily need to be anything huge or complicated. Adding a few simple scents or creating a perfectly chosen playlist can make a big difference. Think about what gets you and your partner excited, and find ways to work those elements into your plans for the night—and keep them handy in your playroom so they are always available.

For each encounter, make it a goal to find a way to stimulate as many senses as possible. For activities where one sense may be compromised —say, when your partner will be blindfolded—make an extra effort to focus on stimulating the other senses, which will be hyperaware at that moment.

After an especially enjoyable encounter together, quiz your partner about the particular sensory stimulants that really stood out for him. Consider this from your own viewpoint, too—what gave you a rush? You might want to jot down a note whenever a specific smell or taste unexpectedly gets you excited, or when the feel of a certain material makes you feel sexy or turned on. These can be clues that help you tune into sensual triggers you may not have noticed before.

Once you start paying attention to these sensory responses and make an effort to stimulate all of your senses, you will wonder how you ever managed to enjoy yourself when you were neglecting some of them. Now, get ready to enjoy a Five Senses Sexual Extravaganza!

Sight

Aside from touch, sight is perhaps the most obvious sense that is involved in sexual experiences, and the pleasure we derive from them. An endless array of visual things can get us excited. You can probably rattle off a whole bunch of them without much thought—seeing your partner showing some skin, seeing her naked (or partially so), watching him pleasure himself or you in some way, and watching her squirm when you get her excited but make her wait for fulfillment.

Then there are sights involving other people that you may find sexually stimulating. This could be watching porn, of course, or it could just be seeing someone you consider appealing. Even just spotting an attractive stranger on the street can be enough to stir your arousal.

But porn is obviously the most common type of sexual visual stimulant. It is also among the easiest to acquire. Thanks to the Internet, you literally have an endless supply of porn at your fingertips 24/7, easily accessible whenever you may feel the urge to look at it. If you prefer a more personal touch, you and your partner could exchange racy e-mails complete with some provocative photos—or even videos, if you have that capability.

You could go with the standard, old-fashioned type of porn: magazines and movies. Both can be very effective, and you can probably find some great options that cater to just about any fetish or turn-on that you and your partner prefer. Take turns picking out the type of porn you will watch or look at. Or pick out a special movie as a surprise for your partner.

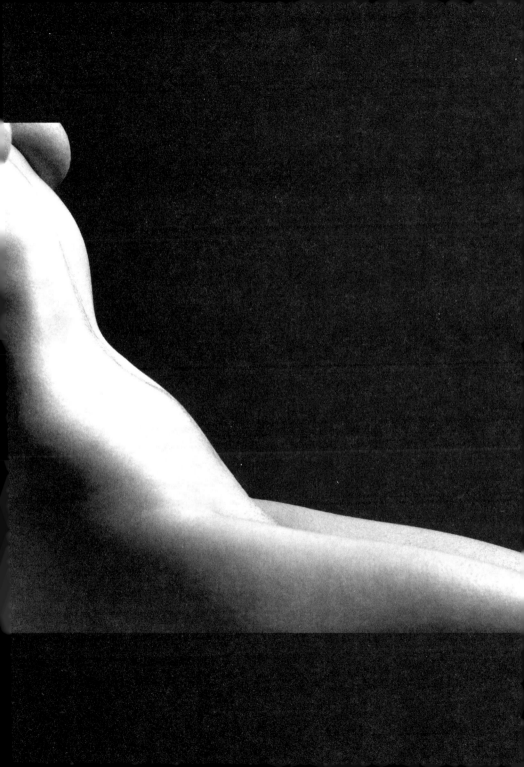

Try to find inspiration or ideas in the porn you enjoy. Look for examples of things you two can act out together, perhaps while adding your own tantalizing twist. Here's another idea: Host your own hot movie festival. Pick your favorite erotic movies and act out a steamy scene from one film each night for a week. You will feel like sexy adult film stars!

Kinky Tip

Here's a way to make watching porn even more exciting: Devise your own adult movie ratings system. You could try a "four stars" type of ratings system or something more complex. Maybe you will assign a certain number of points for each act of penetration, each different sex toy, or whatever. You and your partner will enjoy sharing this inside joke when trying to decide which adult movie to buy or watch.

If you are the dominant, you may want to order your submissive to watch some porn that is a super turn-on for you—and then tell him in detail how you are going to do some of those same acts to him in a few moments. Use the porn as a sort of preview, a sneak peek of what the sub will be in for later that night. This will help get him or her shaky with excitement and anticipation.

But then again, who needs porn when you have a submissive you can order to submit to your wildest desires and demands? Direct your submissive to do something that will be visually exciting to you. The options are practically limitless. You can have her do a striptease. You can instruct him to get naked and pleasure himself. You can use some of your favorite toys on your partner or position her in a way that excites you.

How about going for something more creative or offbeat? Maybe you can incorporate something from one of your fantasies. For example, if you fantasize about nurses, you may order your lover to walk around your house all day dressed in a nurse's uniform—or up the ante and make her walk around in public that way, while you watch from a distance.

Another option: work in a teasing element. Come up with ways to get your partner hot solely by using visual stimulation. Don't allow any sound, touching, or other sensory stimulation. See how crazy you can drive your partner just by providing him with erotic visuals.

Smell

One of our most powerful and sensitive senses is smell. Cleopatra is said to have perfumed the sails of her ship when she went to visit her lover, Marc Antony. An enjoyable smell—or one that evokes a pleasant image or memory—can trigger excitement and arousal. When creating your playroom or sex area, pay special attention to the scents you want to include.

Perfumes and other aromatics have been used for thousands of years, possibly to mimic pheromones—chemicals the body naturally gives off or a signal to some sort of reaction or stimulant.

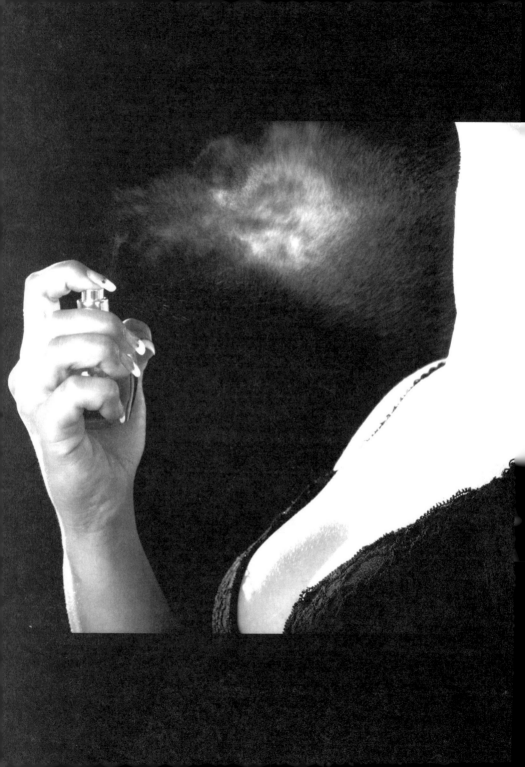

Scent can help you ramp up the sensory excitement of your intimate experiences—and tapping into your olfactory sense is also very easy. You can acquire a wide variety of scents to add to your playroom, without much effort or expense. The exact aroma you want will depend on your preferences and your partner's. Many people enjoy burning incense in their playrooms—incense is available in a wide range of scents and price points. Scented candles are also a good choice—and, as a bonus, candles provide romantic, mood lighting that can enhance your erotic environment and experiences.

 Kinky Tip

One of the most popular scents for lovemaking is musk, which has a smell very close to the male hormone testosterone. Vanilla, lavender, and other floral fragrances have been used for thousands of years to add allure to our bodily scents. Many of the tropical forests in Hawaii were cut down in the eighteenth and nineteenth centuries to produce the delicate musky, earthy scent of sandalwood. The finest European fans for aristocratic women were made from sandalwood. This wood never loses its scent, so it served as a perfume when a woman seductively fanned herself. Fan the flames in your own erotic environment, by wafting your favorite sensual scent throughout your sexy space.

Flowers are also a good way to make your sexy space smell wonderful. The scents of food can also spark your sensory awareness. Cooking can create all sorts of aromas that can help get your pulse racing. Use the trigger system to awaken lascivious memories. Cook a meal that you and your partner enjoyed at a particular romantic dinner, or as a prelude to a really hot night.

When choosing a perfume, pick something that isn't too overbearing. It should compliment the subtle scent of your own skin, hair, and pheromones. Try going without perfume sometimes, especially before a night of sex. This goes for men, too. Don't always wear cologne, which can overpower your own natural erotic smells.

For millennia, incense has been used to enhance sexual environments. Early geishas were said to use incense to help with their seduction techniques. (This may be something to keep in mind for role-playing.) Again, pick something that is appropriate and enticing for you, but is not overbearing—we all have our individual preferences. You might want to place the incense in a special burner in an adjacent room, like a bathroom—especially if you're bothered by smoke—so that the hint of fragrance reaches you rather than its full strength overwhelming you.

Kinky Tip

Be willing to try variety when it comes to scents. Alternate the scents in your romantic environment, trying a different one each night for a week. Note the results in order to determine which scents you do and don't find erotic.

When evaluating the effectiveness of scent, don't rely only on your nose. Yes, it is great if something seems pleasing to your olfactory organs. But scents often trigger chemical reactions or subtle effects that we may not even be consciously aware of. So you may need to be more observant in order to detect the less obvious—yet very powerful—effects of certain scents. Take note of any sudden, unexpected rushes of feelings or intense reactions that may be unusual and can possibly be traced back to the new scent(s) you have added to the mix.

When it comes to scents, don't be afraid to consider new and different options. You might be surprised at what types of scents get some people excited. One recent study found that the smell of black licorice tended to get men aroused. So be creative!

If both of you are addicted to chocolate, try burning some chocolate-scented candles in your love nest. Or create your own makeshift perfume by placing a dish of melted chocolate near a slowly turning fan. Perhaps the two of you have great memories of your recent X-rated romp on a tropical beach. In that case, a simple whiff of suntan lotion might be all it takes to get things rolling. Many women joke that the smell of broiling steak is a major turn-on for their men. Go with whatever works.

Other ideas include:

- Dabbing perfume or essential oils on various body parts, especially erogenous zones
- Pouring essential oils in your bath water to help you enjoy a relaxing soak before your sex play, or when you will be enjoying a sexy bath for two
- Using oils for full-body massages, or even just for foot rubs

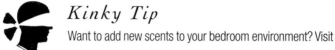

Kinky Tip

Want to add new scents to your bedroom environment? Visit an aromatherapy store and check out the wide variety of scented oils, candles, lotions, and other sensory treats they have to offer. You will most likely discover several new exciting scents that will be the perfect addition to your space. Some fragrance establishments can even help you concoct your own unique blend—which may end up becoming your special signature "sex scent."

Keep in mind: just as good scents can make the sex great, bad scents can totally kill the mood. After all, it is very tough to be romantic if an unpleasant smell is wafting through the air. Be sure to keep your "pleasure room" clean and scrubbed, and be alert for any strange or unpleasant smells that might spoil the experience.

Touch

Touch is, of course, the most obvious sense involved in sexual experiences. There is no end to the possible ways you can turn each other on through various types of touching. Humans crave touching, and the benefits of skin-to-skin contact are well known. A study of married couples by researchers at Brigham Young University and the University of Utah found that massage and gentle touching lowered stress hormones and blood pressure, while also boosting oxytocin, a hormone believed to help alleviate stress.

Before we even get to skin-to-skin contact, though, pay attention to the other things in your sexy space that will be touching you and/ or your partner. Let's start with the obvious: your sheets. Good sheets can make a huge difference in the overall sensual experience of love-making. Many people feel sexy when lying on silk or satin sheets. But depending on the mood you are trying to set, you may want to opt for a different material. The main thing is to invest in at least one set of really good sheets.

But don't fall into the trap of wanting to protect your good sheets. Sure, you may have spent a pretty penny on them—but look at it as an investment in your sexual happiness. Don't be afraid to get them messy. When it comes to sheets, it's usually true that the messier they are, the more fun you are having. Go wild—you can always wash the sheets later.

You may want to incorporate other materials into your playroom décor. Leather is one popular choice. Fur, or fake fur, is an erotic, animalistic turn-on for many people.

But what about the most exciting type of touch—the touch of skin while you and your partner are in close intimate contact? That's perhaps the most important touch—and possibly the most important sensual stimulation—of all. Frankly, you don't even need to do much to make this exciting. Just the fact that you are sharing a sexy or romantic moment and are enjoying this close personal contact will probably get your partner aroused.

However, to up the ante, touch your partner in an especially tender or exciting way. Try running your finger along the skin of a sensitive area—along her spine, say, or upper thigh. Use a very light, featherlike

touch—or use a feather, if you like. This will send shivers through your lover's body.

Add some warming massage oil to the mix while you rub down your partner—it will literally heat up her reaction and the experience.

Want to know exactly how your partner likes to be touched? Just ask him. Pay attention to clues, too. Most likely it will be very obvious when you are touching your lover in a way that he or she really likes. Do some research into acupressure to learn about points on the body that are especially sensitive or associated with sexuality. Then make it a point to focus on these areas during a sensual massage—it will really help get your partner aroused!

Taste

Your tongue has thousands of taste buds, tiny receptors that process the flavor of foods and send messages to your brain. Taste can play a role in your sexual pleasure in numerous ways. The most intimate way is when your tongue savors the taste of your partner. This can occur through any sort of mouth-to-skin contact—through kissing, of course, and oral sex. Just as your partner's scent can trigger a chemical reaction for you, so too can his or her taste.

Let you partner know how good he tastes and how much you enjoy having his special flavor on your lips and tongue. Tell her exactly what she tastes like and how delicious her unique personal flavor is. Better yet, let your actions do the talking and demonstrate just how turned on you are by her taste.

Edible Aphrodisiacs

We've all heard the stories about aphrodisiacs and their supposedly magical libido-boosting powers. Nobody can say for sure whether certain foods actually do affect you biologically—but it's fun to give them a try.

Conduct your own aphrodisiac test run. This is a fun (and tasty!) experiment to try. Make a list of all the foods you can think of that are supposedly aphrodisiacs. Spend a week (or longer, if needed) incorporating one of these foods into your meal every day or night. Monitor the results and see which ones turn up the heat for you, and which simply leave a bad taste in your mouth. It's like having your own sexy test kitchen! Here are some rumored aphrodisiacs to try:

- Oysters: Oysters are perhaps the most well-known of all stereotypical aphrodisiacs. Even if you do not particularly like eating oysters, try sampling them at least once to see if they really live up to the hype.
- Chocolate: In addition to all of its other great qualities, many people believe chocolate can help put you in the mood for romance. As an added bonus, chocolate is so versatile—you can eat it as is, drip it on other foods, or use it to decorate each other's bodies.

- Liquor: Liquor (especially champagne and wine) is also high on the list of alleged aphrodisiacs. Wine adds a romantic feeling to an event and makes even a boring dinner more exciting. Plus, alcohol helps you relax and shed your inhibitions.
- Spices: Some spices reportedly have libido-boosting qualities, including nutmeg and ginger. Try a few combinations and see if you can add some spice to your sex life—literally. You can just mix some spices at random, or check a cookbook for ideas as to some tasty combinations.
- Garlic: Although garlic gets a bad rap for tainting your breath, some people claim garlic is an aphrodisiac. It helps to increase the body's circulation—and enhanced blood flow to certain areas is essential for good sex.

Just about anything can be an aphrodisiac in the right situation. Remember the rumors about green M&M's? It may be hard to believe, but even arugula has been reported to have aphrodisiac qualities.

But why rely on other people's research? Make a conscious effort to see how certain foods affect your level of sexual interest. Pay attention to the food–libido connection and see if you can identify your own unique turn-on foods. Aphrodisiacs need not be exotic or expensive. For some people, cheap junk food does the trick, and you might discover that steak puts your meat-and-potatoes man in the mood. Sometimes it's not just the food itself that does the trick—it's a psychological connection, especially if a certain food triggers the memory of an exciting experience from the past.

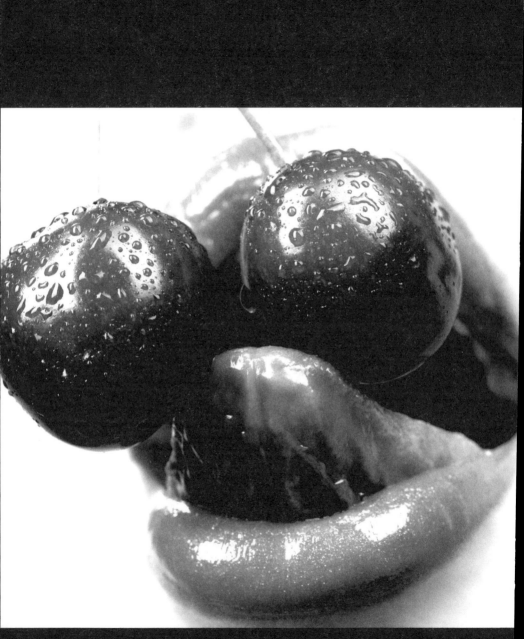

Don't Just Eat—Put on a Show

When it comes to food and sex, it's not just about what you eat, it's how you go about eating it. Even ordinary food can seem sexy if you put a little effort into how you eat or present it.

Make it sexy. Putting any type of food in your mouth can be sexy, if you do it right. No matter what you happen to be eating, make an effort to put a sexy spin on the process. Lick it very slowly, caressing the food with your lips. Really take your time and enjoy it.

Amaze your partner with your cherry skills. Try to master the fine art of tying a cherry stem into a knot using your tongue. This will take some practice, but it is a skill that will impress your partner and make her fantasize about what else you can do with your talented tongue. (Plus it's a great party trick!)

Use your body as a serving tray. Sure, you can feed your lover in all sorts of sexy ways, but few approaches are more erotic (not to mention more direct) than using your own body as a table or serving tray. In the Japanese dining art called Nyotaimori, sushi or sashimi is served on the naked body of a woman. Lie down on the floor, table, or other flat (and sturdy) surface and set out a fun feast on yourself—making sure it's nothing too hot for comfort. To increase the mouth-to-skin contact, place the food directly on your body without any plates or trays. This will force your partner to lick the food from your skin. (Warning: this will also increase the messiness, especially if your meal involves sticky foods.)

To make things more exciting, try the "eating off someone's body" technique while blindfolded. You will need to feel your way around your partner's anatomy for the food, which will make things more fun.

Another fun twist: Make a game out of your sexy meal by requiring your partner to come up with a creative way to incorporate each food item into erotic foreplay. Sure, it's easy with stuff like whipped cream—but requires real imagination in the case of food items like, say, spaghetti.

Here are some other ideas for making food part of your sexy foreplay:

- Use food as a roadmap. Use whipped cream, chocolate, or other edible treats to give your partner a little guidance. Put the food on parts of your body you want your partner to lick, touch, or otherwise pay attention to. He will appreciate the hints—and will also enjoy watching you apply the food to your hot spots.
- Make an edible erotic combination. Put half of your "recipe" on your own body, and the other half on your partner's, then rub together to create the perfect tasty blend. For example, you can wear the chocolate syrup while he wears the cherries.
- Do a private taste test when you're out with your partner taking care of mundane things—getting groceries or picking up supplies at the hardware store. When no one's looking, slip a finger into your panties and then touch it to his tongue. Do that a few times to tease him. When you get home, get out of those panties and push his head between your legs.
- Give him a citrus shower. Bend an orange slice until it bursts and sprays his penis. The citrus juice will send a refreshingly cool sensation over him. This would also work with a slice of lemon or lime.

- Give her a cherry tickler. Tickle her clitoris or nipples with a cherry stem. Be careful that the ends are not too sharp. For an added twist, dip the stem in chocolate or liquor beforehand, and then lick up the trail it leaves behind.
- Drink hot (but not too hot) tea while performing oral sex. The warm liquid—coupled with the warmth of your mouth—will give your partner an extra thrill. Alternate between warm and chilled drinks, to provide both sensations of heat and cold.

Sound

Sound is another important aspect of creating a great sexual space. Just as most of the greatest movies have memorable soundtracks, we often add our own mental soundtrack to important moments in our lives.

Music

The right background music can help ensure you have the perfect ambience for your bedroom action. Music helps set the mood and can even be used to help choreograph the evening's progression of sexual activities.

You probably already have a favorite repertoire of music that you and your partner have used in the past, with sexual success. Great! Keep using those songs as much as you like—the precedent will prompt you to mentally connect that wonderful feeling with the music. As soon as you hear the first few notes, your pulse may immediately start racing.

But continue adding to your passion playlist, to keep things new and exciting and allow yourself to enjoy some new auditory experiences.

If you and your partner like different types of music, take turns creating a mix of both. Of course, the dominant person may assume the power to control the music most of the time, but perhaps he could grant the submissive the opportunity to choose the tunes occasionally as a reward for good behavior.

If you have the ability to record, try creating a whole love-track of music especially for your sex play. Have enough songs prepared to last for an erotic evening that may be several hours long. You could even create several different tracks, each designed especially for a certain type of activities—say, one for massage, one for the dominant to control his sex slave, etc.

A recent trend incorporates classical music into sex—there can be something exciting about combining this highbrow, sophisticated type of music with physical activities that are so raw, basic, and primitive. And many people find this type of music soothing. Plus, a lot of people find they prefer instrumental music for intimate interludes—lyrics can be distracting and you don't want to get caught singing along when you should be focused on more important things. If you are aiming for a peaceful mood, you may even want to look for a CD that plays sounds of the ocean or the forest. On the other hand, music with a driving beat can get your blood pumping.

Choosing the right soundtrack can really affect your romantic intensity. Some people like to adjust the music selections depending on the specific sensual activity they have planned. During foreplay, for example, you might select music specifically designed for meditation or yoga, to encourage a leisurely relaxing pace.

Although your musical tastes may vary, here are some sexy suggestions to get you started. (Tip: for inspiration, go to a strip club. Strippers have a knack for picking sexy music that tends to have the kind of throbbing beat that gets your blood pumping.)

- "Strut" by Sheena Easton. The name says it all.
- "You Shook Me All Night Long" by AC/DC. It is impossible not to strut your stuff with that song blaring.
- "Pour Some Sugar on Me" by Def Leppard. Every stripper has this song in her rotation.
- "Talk Dirty to Me" by Poison. Because it's just so damn appropriate.
- "Wild Thing" by Tone Loc. There is no question what this song is about, and it is almost impossible to sit still when you hear it.
- "I Touch Myself" by the Divinyls. Another very clear message. Play this while talking to your partner on the phone. Ask, "Can you guess what I am doing?"

Musical tastes may vary, but few people enjoy getting romantic in total silence. At the very least, you might want to invest in a white noise machine to help block out the racket from the outside world.

Vocal Sounds and Commands

We can't really fully discuss the sounds of sex (or the sounds that accompany or encourage sex) without talking about . . . well, talking. Or any types of noise that we make with our own mouths.

One of the sexiest sounds your partner can hear in bed is the sound of your own voice. It doesn't even need to be a sexy voice (although that certainly wouldn't hurt). Just hearing you say something, anything, is better than silence.

Vocal noise takes on a somewhat unique meaning in a BDSM arrangement because this situation often involves—perhaps even requires—one partner (the dominant) to take an authoritative tone of voice with the other. By definition, a dominant must be powerful and in charge. That means it is necessary to give commands, possibly in a stern and cold manner. Even if this doesn't come naturally to you, it's important to master this art because it will help your submissive know that you are in charge, and will convey that your orders are to be followed. It may take a little bit of time and practice for you to become comfortable giving orders to your partner in a convincing and effective way.

Of course, we're all familiar with other types of vocal sounds connected to sex. Moaning and yelling, for example. Some people are just quieter by nature. But if you really want your partner to get more vocal, you could include that in one of your commands, if you are the dominant. Order him to yell and swear—tell him exactly what to say and then make him repeat it, perhaps several times if he isn't totally convincing the first time.

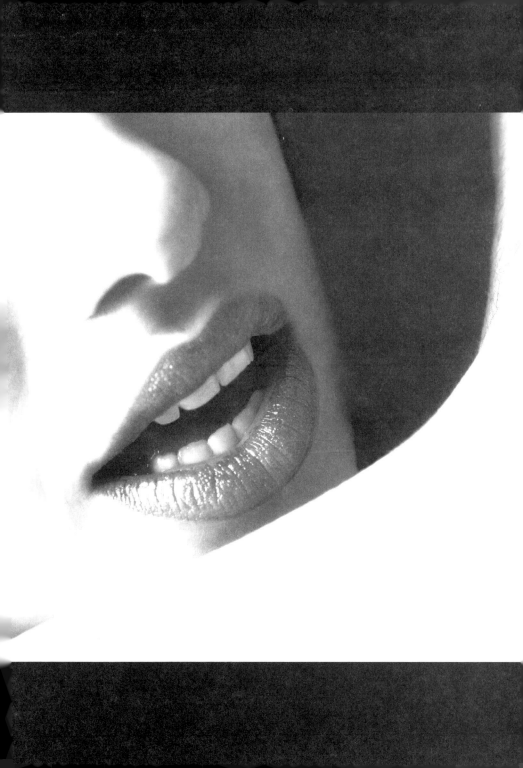

It can be very sexy to hear your partner tell you what she wants you to do to her. Tease your partner by withholding the action you know she wants, until she requests it in either a proper and respectful way (or perhaps begging) or a commanding and forceful way, depending on what you are looking for.

Hold up your end of the bargain, too. People (especially men) often complain that they do not know how to please their partners because they are clueless as to what their partners want. Don't leave it up to guesswork. Tell your partner exactly what you want. No long-winded explanation is needed. A simple, "Put your tongue there—now!" should do the trick. If you suspect your partner may be unsure what to do to turn you on, this can help give him clear-cut directions.

On the opposite side, it can also be very erotic (and deliciously torturous) to spell out exactly what you plan to do to your partner. Announce in very specific and graphic terms just what you are going to do each step of the way. This will likely be a huge turn-on for both of you, and will really have your partner quaking in anticipation.

Tip: saying (or shouting) your partner's name in the throes of passion can be a turn-on for him, especially as part of a sensual utterance like, "Oh, Rick, that drives me crazy—it feels so good!" Your partner will know you are totally focused on him.

One of the biggest turn-offs for people of both genders is a partner who is too quiet in bed. We all want to have clear evidence that we are pleasing our partners and the easiest and most effective way to demonstrate that is by making lots of noises that broadcast exactly how much fun you are having. So don't be shy—do lots of moaning, yelling, cursing, sighing, and any other types of verbal encouragement you wish to express. Make your pleasure known loud and clear.

Kinky Tip

If you aren't normally the type to utter four-letter words, suddenly letting loose with a couple can really get your partner's attention. Turn the dirty talk on, and you will probably turn your partner on, in a big way. If you are usually more timid, hearing you utter naughty words like "pussy" and "cock" will not only make your partner take notice but it will also make it clear to him that you are really excited and getting caught up in the spirit of the action. Even better, learn some new words. Watch a few new porn movies or read some adult magazines to brush up on your sexy slang. Bust out a few dirty words your partner has never heard you use before.

Chapter 7

Tie Me Up: Restraints and Harnesses

"It is always by way of pain
one arrives at pleasure."

—Marquis de Sade

Once you've established a level of trust with your lover and are ready to introduce another delicious experience to your sex play, it's time to try being restrained. You don't have to do anything drastic right away. Allow your dom to gently ease you into the titillating world of restraints and harnesses. The idea of being "restrained" can take many forms, from a loosely wrapped necktie to chains and handcuffs. In other words, it can be a mostly symbolic gesture that allows you to easily free yourself quickly—or a more intense situation in which you are unable to escape on your own.

In this chapter, we will cover a range of sexual activities that relate to being tied up. In other words, we will boldly explore the world of bondage or the "B" in BDSM.

Many people find bondage exciting, for a variety of reasons. Just the physical feeling of being restrained or held back from touching their lovers or themselves can often be stimulating. Giving over total control or having it (depending on which role you take) is also sexually thrilling and can deepen the sensual bond with your partner.

Being tied up is a basic staple of bondage activities. Here we'll explore a wide spectrum of specific sexual activities, ranging from mild to extreme. Though you may not take the formal step of putting things in writing, it might be a good idea to at least have a quick chat about what you are comfortable with, and where you draw the line. If you are just starting out with the relatively tame practice of wrapping a necktie loosely around the wrists, this may not require a specific conversation. But for more advanced or confining forms of restraint, it's probably a good idea to establish your limits beforehand.

Many people start very gradually when it comes to sexual activities that involve being tied up. Often, it begins with a fun, casual move that may be totally unplanned—such as taking off the scarf or tie your partner is wearing and using it to tease or seduce your lover in the course of a romantic encounter. But you might discover being tied up is a turn-on for you, and you may decide to escalate your play to include other forms of bondage. You can then build the sexual tension and excitement by gradually increasing the role and type of bondage in your play activities. It can also be fun to locate creative new bondage supplies and toys to add to your playroom "treasure chest."

Neckties and Plastic Ties

When it comes to restraints, neckties are probably one of the most popular choices. For one thing, they are easily accessible—found in almost every man's closet. And if you are in the process of getting undressed, you or your partner may be shedding a tie at that moment. Ties seem innocent—you can buy them at your favorite department store without any fear of embarrassment. Likewise, you don't need to hide them if someone shows up at your home expectedly.

If you are new to the idea of being tied up, neckties are a great way to ease into this form of play. Neckties don't look too scary—and you can add to the sexiness factor by slowly removing the tie from around your partner's neck. Or if you are the one sporting the tie, make a tantalizing show of slowly undoing and removing it.

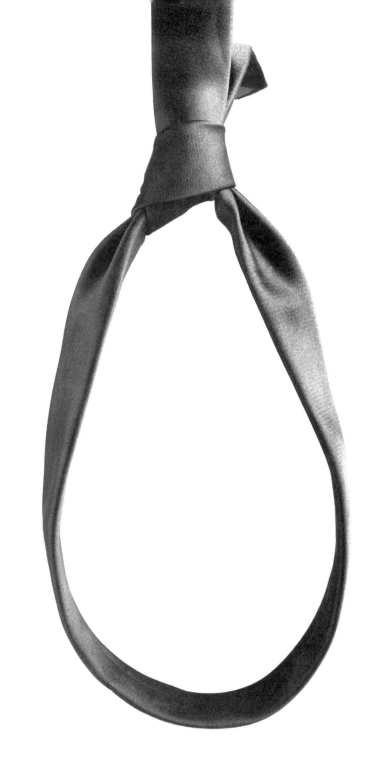

Ladies, you can ramp up the sexual tension by removing your partner's tie and putting it on yourself—while wearing nothing else, ideally. Draw out the moment by slowly running the tie over various parts of your undressed body—the silky fabric feels luscious.

When you are first starting out, you may feel more comfortable with your wrists and/or ankles simply tied together, perhaps with your wrists above your head. This way you can still move your arms/legs if needed. When you feel ready, you can move on to being tied to a bedpost or other object, which will keep you more restrained (and may be a little more scary, yet exciting).

Safe Is Sexy

Be careful not to tie the necktie too tightly when using it as a restraint. It should be loose enough that the person is not in pain. Especially when first trying this, couples often barely secure the tie, so that the "restrained" person could easily remove her hands/feet if she wanted to. This might be more comfortable if the submissive is still getting used to the idea of being tied up. It can also come in handy when you need to remove yourself from the tied-up state quickly.

A nice bonus about incorporating neckties or other seemingly innocent articles of clothing such as scarves into your sex play is that they can become an intimate inside joke between you and your partner. For example, while you are out on a dinner date, your partner may began fiddling with his tie—the very one you were tied up with the night before—and this can serve as a secret turn-on for both of you that nobody else knows about. You can also send each other discreet signals using this prop as a little teaser about what the night's activities may hold.

Using more restrictive forms of ties, such as plastic cable ties, is often scarier for the restrained person as it is difficult (if not impossible) to free yourself without help. It's important to make sure the person in the submissive role is comfortable with this—if so, it can be sexually exciting for both of you. You can find these types of ties at most home improvement stores or supermarkets. You may want to opt for the longer varieties that enable you to bind both hands or both feet simultaneously.

Safe Is Sexy

Plastic ties tend to become tighter when you move or resist, which may be uncomfortable or even painful. If you relax your hands/feet, the tie will likely loosen and be more comfortable. Also, keep in mind that plastic is susceptible to heat, so when using plastic ties keep a safe distance from candles or other heat sources to avoid the risk of burns.

Ropes

Natural filament rope is a good choice for bondage because it is rougher and discourages struggling (or at least makes it more sadistically

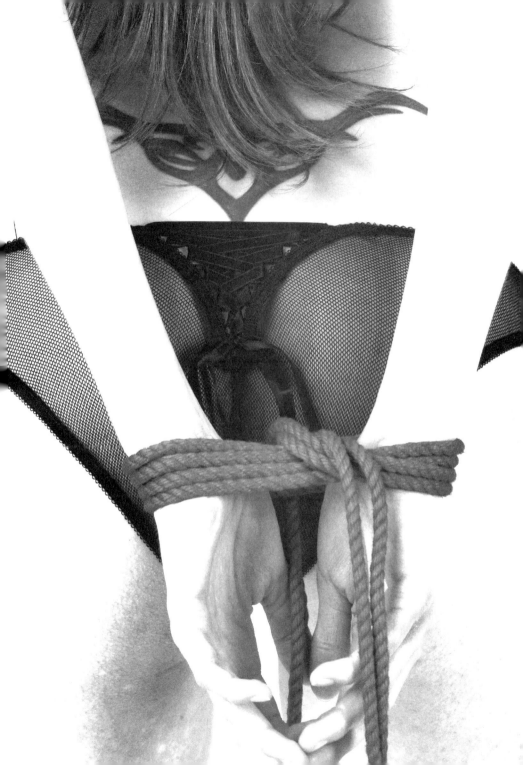

painful). But you can experiment with different types of rope materials to see which ones you and your partner prefer.

Rope is considered a traditional piece of bondage equipment. It can be used by itself to tie someone up, but is also used as part of more complicated suspension or restraint setups.

It might be true that rope is no longer trendy among the bondage scene, though. Some people view it as too old-fashioned or just plain difficult to work with, and have replaced it with sexier and more convenient options, such as fur cuffs or more flexible bonds.

If you do use ropes, be careful and alert to the possibility of rope burns, which can be painful and may be obvious for a while after the rope is removed.

Interesting note: rope made from hemp is a part of traditional Japanese bondage routines, and has become more popular and trendy in the West.

Soft Cuffs and Metal Handcuffs

Cuffs are a common item in adult playrooms and bondage setups, and are often attached to parts of the bed or used as part of a suspension or restraint system. The use of cuffs can be especially exciting when combined with other forms of sexy play, such as blindfolds and spanking. Cuffs may be made from a variety of materials, including fur or leather. They may also be made from metal, which, of course, tends to be more uncomfortable and restrictive.

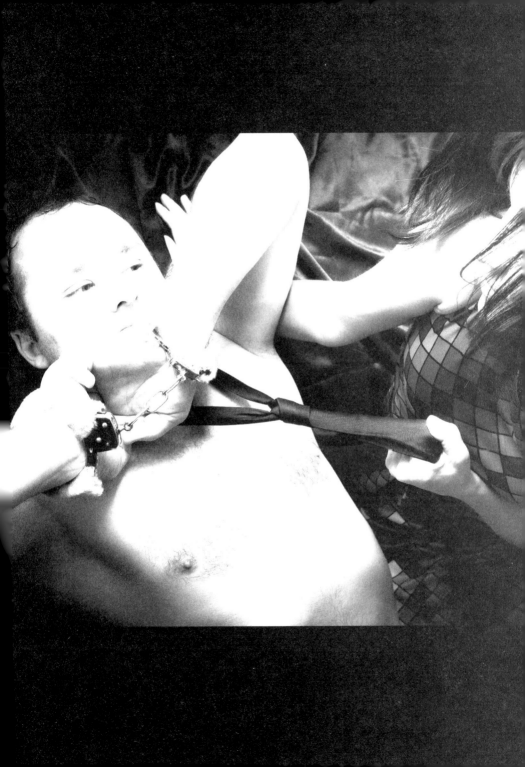

Many people find the idea of handcuffs exciting as part of a fantasy, although some are nervous about taking that step in reality. You will probably be using handcuffs made of a soft material that are specifically designed for fun, as opposed to the type law enforcement officials slap on criminals. There should be a way for the submissive person to release himself if he wants to.

Although metal handcuffs can be intimidating at first, they can also heighten the sexual excitement. Some people find metal handcuffs add a more intense element to their bondage play. But metal cuffs are definitely a matter of personal taste. Some people find the cold steel exhilarating, whereas others find the cuffs painful and prone to pinching skin.

These handcuffs can lock, which may add an extra thrill (or element of danger) to the experience. You can incorporate the process of locking the handcuffs into your play. And, of course, you could also hide the key somewhere or use it as a reward your partner has to earn.

Kinky Tip

To up the ante and add an extra element of excitement, try working the handcuffs into a fantasy scenario. You could pretend to be a cop arresting a criminal, or a spy interrogating a prisoner. Be creative and have fun coming up with all sorts of crimes—and punishments the dom can impose on the submissive.

Spreader Bars and X-Crosses

A spreader bar is a piece of equipment that consists of a metal or wooden bar with cuffs that attach to a person's hands and/or feet. The spreader bar may also have a hanging apparatus so that it can be suspended or affixed to a wall or ceiling. Spreader bars are often used as part of a suspension grid, discussed later.

As you can probably guess from the name, a spreader bar spreads the arms or legs apart. The spreader bar can also be used to keep someone in a spread-eagle position, or just to keep hands and/or feet from moving. The bar prevents the submissive from instinctively tensing up or clenching and closing the legs. It can also secure a person's hands and feet behind the back.

Spreader bars are usually adjustable, so you can change the distance between hands/legs to whatever is comfortable or exciting for you. The bars usually include cuffs and have places to attach other types of bondage equipment. When used to secure both the hands and feet, spreader bars can render a person totally submissive.

If you already have cuffs or other accessories, it would probably be fairly easy to make your own basic spreader bar using a piece of wood or plastic.

A large cross (a crisscross or X-shaped structure) is commonly found in sex playrooms or dungeons. The bondage cross is usually made from wood or metal in the shape of an X. It is sometimes referred to as a St. Andrew's cross or an X-frame cross. Generally attached to a wall, it is sometimes designed to allow for movement and rotation,

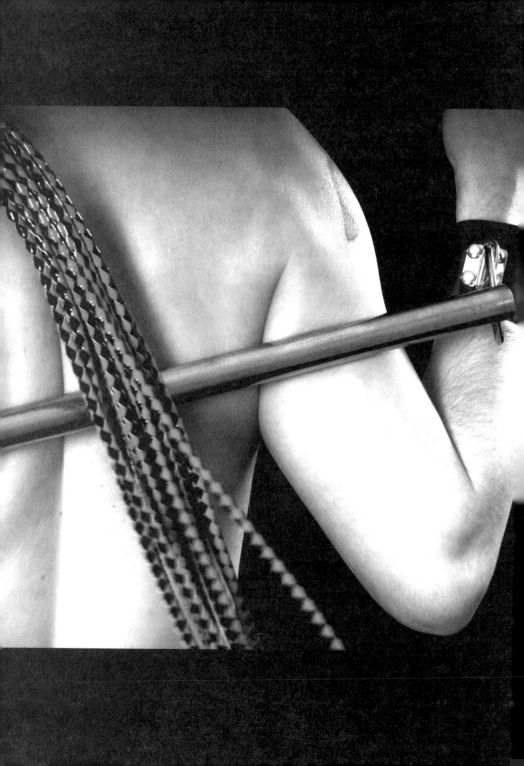

so the person attached to it can be spun around. Make sure it is affixed securely!

Interesting trivia: this structure is nicknamed the St. Andrew's cross because St. Andrew was said to have been crucified on a cross in the shape of an X, rather than the more typical cross depicted in a T shape.

The X-cross allows the wrists and ankles to be secured with cuffs or ties, attaching the submissive in a spread-eagle position. If the person is secured with his face against the cross, he's in a good position for spanking or flogging. For intercourse, the person is usually positioned with her back against the cross.

If you want to try out the X-cross, first make sure the cross is secure and safe. Also, be sure you are comfortable with this level of bondage—and, most likely, submission. You will be in a vulnerable position and won't have much control or ability to move.

Note: if the cross is set up to rotate or spin, it might also be a good idea to start out gradually to make sure you aren't prone to motion sickness or dizzy spells.

Suspension and Suspension Grids

Suspension involves being tied up or restrained and lifted (at least partially) off the ground. The person's body (or parts of it) is suspended using ropes, chains, or some sort of similar apparatus. Suspension systems generally use a type of cuffs that are specifically designed to be more comfortable for someone who is hanging in the air.

Suspension can take a variety of different forms. The person may just be lying down with one or both legs suspended in the air. Or the submissive can be totally suspended—completely lifted off the ground.

The suspension aspect not only adds a level of excitement for one or both partners, but also gives the dominant partner more control, because the submissive has limited—perhaps very little—ability to move freely. Suspension ramps up the risk in a bondage scenario, because it makes the submissive more physically helpless and vulnerable. This, of course, adds to the sexual excitement—at least for the dominant. It can also be dangerous if not used carefully, so it is important to make sure your suspension equipment is set up properly and employed with caution.

What self-respecting dominator would have a playroom that doesn't include a suspension grid? The iron suspension grid can be at least eight square feet in size and hang from the ceiling right in the middle of the room. You might have to work up to using one as some people find it too intense and frightening. This may be something you want to consider as a "soft limit" in your contract. A suspension grid involves a frame sort of structure that is suspended from the ceiling or another structure. It features cuffs, ropes, chains, and/or other elements to allow a person to be suspended for bondage activities.

Like the X-cross, the suspension grid involves some commitment (not to mention effort and planning). You probably won't encounter this apparatus in the home of someone who is new to bondage or is just dabbling in or experimenting with the BDSM lifestyle. This piece of equipment is more likely to show up in a full-scale, totally outfitted playroom—or a sex club or dominatrix studio.

As with the X-cross, it is exactly because the suspension grid is less common that some people find it to be exciting—or at least intriguing —when they have the opportunity to encounter one and try it out. Even if it isn't the kind of thing you want to do every day, it might be fun for an occasional adventure.

The Bottom Line on Bondage

As you can see, bondage can run the gamut from mild to wild, with lots of variations (and logistical scenarios) in between. If you are curious about bondage—or just want to add something new to your restraint repertoire—there are lots of options, and lots of equipment and accessories you can try, including many you can easily locate in your own closets or buy at a mainstream store. You can surely find a few that suit your tastes and comfort level.

Chapter 8

Punish Me: Methods for When You've Been Bad

"I was often very, incredibly naughty, and if I didn't come home at tea time I used to be sent to bed without any dinner. But people used to bring me things: I was better fed in bed."

— Diane Cilento

A big part of the BDSM approach to sex is the idea of control and power. The dominant has the power and sets the rules (once the initial rules have been spelled out in the contract or agreement). To maintain control, the dominant must order the submissive to follow the rules and make sure they are enforced. Obviously, this means there must be consequences when the rules are not followed or the submissive does not behave in a way that is pleasing or satisfying to the dominant.

In other words, there must be punishment.

Now, we are all familiar with the concept of punishment. Most of us have had experience with that (perhaps lots of it) from when we were children. Those of you who are parents have also experienced the other side of the punishment scenario, having to dole out punishment for your children. Punishment in that sense is never fun, either for the one receiving it or the one handing it out.

In the BDSM context, punishment has an entirely different meaning. Yes, you are experiencing a negative consequence for "bad behavior." But in this case, the person doling out the punishment is enjoying it. And possibly so is the person receiving it, at least in some way. An important thing to remember is that both people are involved in the punishment process voluntarily, and both agree to it. It is exciting to both parties in some ways, although obviously the specifics can differ for the dominant and the submissive.

In BDSM the actual punishment itself is also very unique. It can take all sorts of forms, including physical actions or verbal reprimands. The exact type of punishment may be specified in (or at least governed by) the contract you have with your partner. But for many couples, part of the excitement is the dominant's ability to decide the punishment and come up with some creative and exciting options.

The most common types of BDSM punishments probably involve something like spanking. However, it is also common for punishment to take the form of disapproval or even a denial of pleasure. In some cases, the punishment may involve the dominant ordering the submissive to abstain from certain pleasurable acts. Then, of course, there are punishments that involve humiliation or embarrassment. This is more common in arrangements where there is a "sex slave" type of scenario.

Hands Only: Spanking, Slapping, and Hitting

Many types of punishment involve the dominant using his hands to inflict physical pain on the submissive. This can take the form of spanking, slapping, or other forms of hitting. The most important thing to remember here is that the dominant is not trying to inflict any sort of serious or permanent harm on the submissive. And again, both parties must agree to the specific type and manner of punishment. This is especially important for the submissive, who must give full consent to the punishment and make sure it doesn't cross the line of what she is comfortable with.

One thing many people like about punishment involving hands is that it can seem intimate and personal, because there is skin-to-skin contact. Also, this allows the dominant to caress the submissive in between the punishing acts.

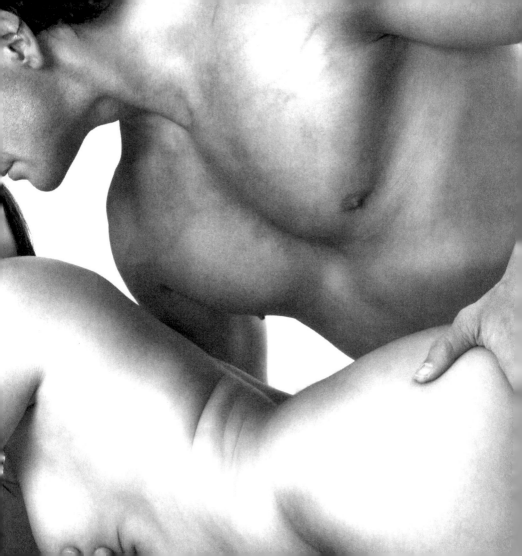

Spanking is probably the most common type of punishment involving the hands. People find spanking exciting for a variety of reasons. For some, the idea that you are a bad child who must be disciplined by an authority figure is appealing. This comes into play when couples act out or adopt a sort of parent-and-child scenario—or perhaps a schoolboy and his teacher.

Another advantage is that spanking offers the opportunity for a lot of variety and can be customized to the parties' individual tastes. First of all, there is the choice of position. The most obvious is the traditional spanking arrangement, with the spanker putting the spankee over his knee. But you can vary this standard position by adjusting the angle and position of the person being spanked. Sometimes the dominant will position the submissive in such a way that the genitals have maximum exposure. This not only affects the physical sensation, but it can also increase the humiliation factor and make the submissive feel more vulnerable.

Another option is to have the submissive stand and bend over, as if he were touching his toes. This puts his ass in a very vulnerable position, and also gives him a different viewpoint from which he can see the dominant approaching from behind. Visually, this position can be exciting for the dominant because she can see the submissive's entire body. Some couples also enjoy a variation where the submissive is kneeling, with her ass resting on her heels or raised up in the air, ready for the dominant to spank it from behind.

The submissive may also have his hands and/or feet bound or restrained while he is in position, to make him more vulnerable and also to prevent him from instinctively covering himself with his hands in a protective action.

To make the spanking more exciting and unexpected, the dominant should make an effort to vary the strength, rhythm, and timing of the spanking sessions. Another way to change up the basic spanking session is with the type and amount of clothing (if any) that each party is wearing. Often the submissive will be totally nude while the dominant is fully clothed, to emphasize the idea that the dominant is in control while the submissive is vulnerable. But sometimes the submissive will just have his or her pants pulled down, to imitate the typical appearance of a child being spanked. It may even be exciting to spank the submissive while she has her panties or something else still on. Or a female submissive could wear a low-cut top and short skirt with no panties underneath.

Kinky Tip

To take spanking or similar types of punishment to the next level, you can buy or make a spanking bench, whipping post, or other type of furniture to use for this purpose. This piece of furniture can also come in handy for other activities—but it is more powerful in a symbolic way if it is used solely for punishment experiences.

Generally the dominant will start slowly and with a relatively mild force, and then increase both the speed and force of his blows as he and his partner become more excited. An important part of the process is the build-up. Once the submissive has assumed the proper position, the dominant slowly assesses her and looks at her entire body. The dominant will approach slowly, allowing the anticipation to build. Often the dominant will then spend some time gently caressing the area that will be spanked or hit. He may even use his finger or mouth to get the submissive aroused prior to the spanking.

Another type of punishment that uses only the hands is slapping, which is often similar to spanking. It is important to use caution and carefully select the areas of the body that will be slapped. Certain areas are much more easily injured and prone to serious damage than others. Soft fleshy areas such as the buttocks are usually the best choice.

The dominant should make an effort to lovingly caress the area of his partner's body that is being spanked or slapped, both in between strikes and when the session is over.

The dominant may also want to use his hands to grab or restrain the submissive, holding them in a forceful way. This is often used in conjunction with some sort of verbal punishment.

Other forms of hitting should probably be discussed and established beforehand. Often, hitting someone with your hand in certain ways can cause negative emotional reactions—even if it is supposed to be part of sex play—and can even closely resemble actions that would happen in an abusive relationship. It's important to explore your partner's feelings in depth and make sure she can handle whatever type of punishment you decide upon. If there is any doubt, it is better to err on the side of caution and choose something else.

Using Crops

To step up the idea of spanking or slapping, the dominant may want to use a crop. This is an item similar to a riding crop used on a horse. It is used to strike the person in a way that usually inflicts a sharp, stinging sensation.

Crops come in many different sizes and styles. Some are small enough to fit in a purse—which can be handy if you want to be able to discipline your submissive in a number of locations.

These crops are also made from a variety of materials, included leather and braided horsehair. The different types of materials result in much different sensations, so it is a good idea to try out a few kinds to see which provides the effect you want. Some styles of crops have something at the "striking" end for added impact. One style features a red leather heart with metal studs. This is sure to add both visual appeal and a unique physical sensation!

One big allure of using a crop is the visual stimulation. It can be exciting for both parties when the dominant pulls out a crop and starts whipping it around (or to build the anticipation, slowly caressing it). And, of course, there is the sound of the crop snapping or hitting skin. That unmistakable sound certainly leaves no doubt as to who is in charge in this situation! The whole picture definitely establishes the authority of the dominant and fits the image of BDSM that many of us have in our minds.

To heighten the submissive's senses, the dominant will often begin by slowly running the crop over her partner's exposed body in a tickling or teasing manner. She may also use the tip of the crop to penetrate

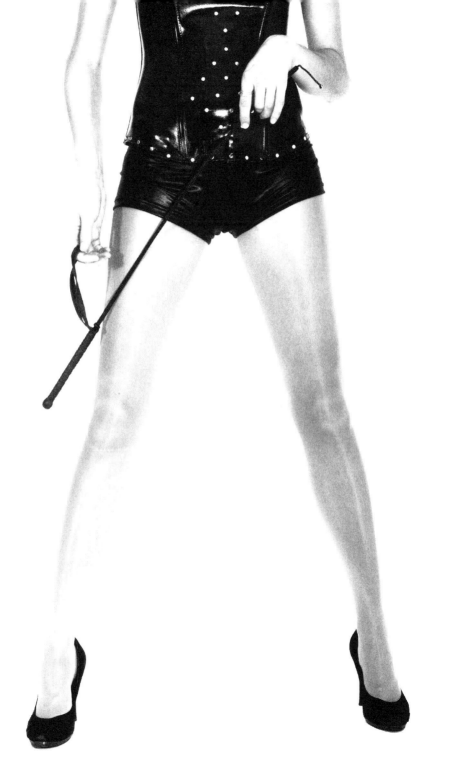

or stimulate her partner. As with many other play toys, this makes the crop an implement the dominant can use to provide an exquisite combination of both pleasure and pain.

A note on caning: caning is similar to using a crop, except a cane is a long thin piece of equipment designed to inflict a sharp and painful sting. Caning can be very painful, especially if the dominant is not experienced with the practice. Many couples do not like to use canes, and it is probably fairly common for this item to be listed in the hard limits section of the contract. Should either you or your partner consider caning, do your research and give this a lot of thought before even considering it.

Flogging

Flogging involves striking a person with a flogger, an instrument that is somewhat similar to a crop, except the striking end contains numerous strips of material—sometimes called "tails"—that are used to hit the person. The flogger is held with a heavily weighted handle, which allows the dominant to control the flogging action and the rhythm and force of the strokes.

Like crops, flogs can be made from a variety of materials. Among the most common are suede and leather. The texture and width of the specific type of material used to make the tails can have a big impact on the feeling of getting hit with the flogger. Some materials are notorious for inflicting a major sting, so try out a few types and see which feels best for you.

As with a crop, when using a flogger it is best to start slowly and gently, and then gradually intensify your force and speed. It can also feel very thrilling if you run the tails of the flogger over sensitive areas of your partner's naked body. The tickling feeling of all of the tails dancing across the quivering skin makes for quite the excitement! Even better if your partner is blindfolded and cannot see what you are doing. Adding the right music can complete the perfect setting for this type of play.

To really maximize the experience, you can use a flogger in each hand. This allows you to maintain a more rapid series of strokes or to strike several different areas of your partner's body. Or you can graze the tip of the flogger on or near your partner's genitals, breasts, or other sensitive areas. This gives her a preview of the action and gives her time to think about what you are going to do to her.

 Kinky Tip

It is a good idea to practice using a crop or flog on a pillow or other inanimate object, to help you get the hang of it before you actually use it on a person. This gives you a chance to become comfortable with how you handle the toy and lets you practice to find the perfect rhythm and technique. Also, some BDSM communities or clubs actually give workshops where you can learn the correct way to use these and other BDSM toys and equipment. Of course, you can also do an online search for video demonstrations.

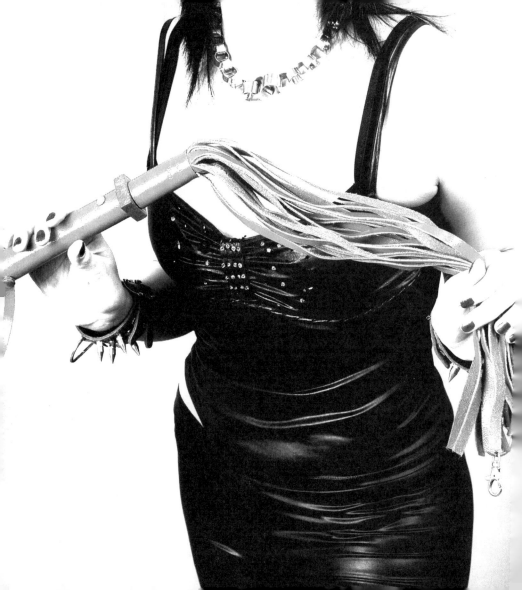

When using a crop or flogger, you usually want to have the submissive restrained—either by using cuffs or ties, or by placing the person on a suspension grid or cross. This keeps the sub from moving around too much, and also makes the experience more visually stimulating to the dominant.

In addition to crops and floggers, paddles are also commonly used to inflict punishment on a submissive. The paddle is used for spanking and adds a different sensation and force than spanking with a hand. Paddles come in many different sizes and are constructed of different types of materials. Some are even covered in fur or other soft material. These paddles are obviously used more for the visual impact of spanking, as opposed to inflicting any sort of actual pain. You could, of course, create your own paddle or use some sort of household object as a makeshift paddle.

Safe Is Sexy

When planning or carrying out any type of punishment, be sure to adhere to the hard limits, but also be alert for any signs of extreme emotional distress. This is especially true if your partner has had an abusive relationship in the past. If so, the act of being physically punished may suddenly cause the submissive to have negative flashbacks or experience an emotional reaction that can be very harmful.

Sometimes the dominant will further torture the submissive by making her choose the instrument for her own punishment. However, this can backfire if any of the items are actually pleasurable to the submissive. In that case, the dominant would want to exclude that item from among the choices.

Anticipation is often incorporated into the punishment process. The submissive may be blindfolded and/or bound and left in silence for some period of time to await his punishment. Sometimes the dominant will also use headphones or earplugs to keep the submissive from hearing any sounds that may be clues as to what is about to happen. During this time, the submissive will be so anxious about the mysterious punishment that all his senses will be hypersensitive and totally alert.

Another option: create a deck of punishment cards. To further torture your submissive, you can force him to create the cards. When the submissive misbehaves, you or the submissive will select one card at random from the deck. This adds to the anticipation of waiting to see what the punishment will be.

Mental and Verbal Punishment

Frequently, BDSM punishment does not involve only physical actions. Often, there will be some verbal aspect to the punishment. This can take many forms. The dominant may simply take a very stern tone with the submissive, thereby punishing her partly by withholding the affection of a gentle tone. This indication of disapproval is a symbolic form of punishment, and can in some ways be more powerful and effective than any physical actions.

The verbal punishment can sometimes be harsher, with the dominant yelling, cursing, or belittling the submissive—possibly calling her names like "slut" or "whore." This is intended to add an aspect of humiliation to the experience—and also to stress the dominant's authority and power.

The verbal punishment can also take a different tactic. The dominant may force the submissive to say certain things. This could mean reciting an admission of his offenses, or begging the dominant for leniency. Or the submissive may be required to say something embarrassing or degrading, for example, yelling, "I am a slut!" or "I am a bad boy who needs to be punished."

This type of punishment often goes hand in hand with mental or psychological punishment. Again, this can take many forms. The dominant may withhold affection (emotional and/or physical) from the submissive. Or the submissive may be prohibited from engaging in any sort of sexual or physical pleasure during the punishment period (we'll talk later about withholding orgasm).

Punishment can also involve some sort of humiliation or "sentence." The submissive may have to do the dominant's household chores or serve as his slave, for example. Or she might have to do something embarrassing.

The submissive may also be deprived of physical contact with the dominant for whatever period of time the punishment lasts. For added discomfort, the dominant may deliberately try to get the submissive aroused, so the inability to satisfy his physical urges will become even more frustrating.

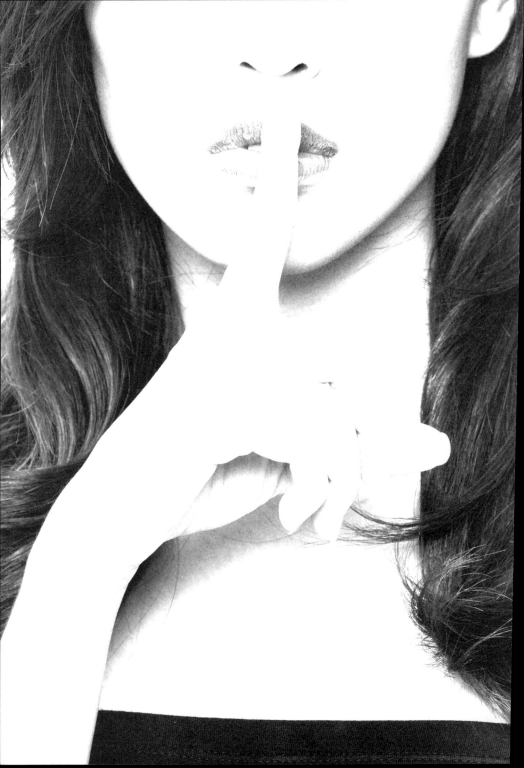

Kinky Tip
Some submissives really do enjoy pain and will deliberately "misbehave" in order to provoke the dominant into punishing them. These submissives are sometimes referred to as "pain sluts" in the BDSM community. In this case, inflicting any sort of physical action such as flogging would only give the submissive what he wants—so if you're the dominant you could punish the submissive by withholding flogging, spanking, or any other physical actions.

Interestingly, one relatively common—and effective—form of punishment in BDSM relationships is to deprive the submissive of the opportunity to serve the dominant. This is mainly the case in arrangements where the submissive acts as a servant or sex slave to the dominant. In these situations, the submissive takes pride in and gets sexual pleasure from serving her "master." Depriving her of this privilege can be a very strong form of punishment.

Withholding Orgasm

A fairly common punishment—and a uniquely agonizing sort of torture—involves preventing the submissive from climaxing. In other words, the dominant withholds the privilege of orgasm from the submissive. This punishment stresses the fact that the dominant has sole power and control over the submissive—specifically, over her physical pleasure and sexual satisfaction.

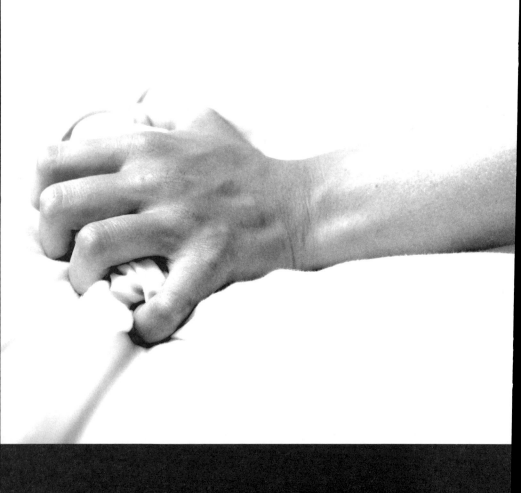

This can mean withholding any sort of sexual pleasure completely. But usually it involves forcing the submissive to be stimulated (or to stimulate himself) to the brink of climax, and then making him stop. This is sometimes referred to as "edging" because the submissive almost reaches the edge of no return, but then is quickly yanked back. The submissive will often reach the point of begging the dominant for permission to climax. This can be extremely frustrating and can sometimes reach the point where it is physically painful. To further torture the submissive, the dominant may repeatedly climax in front of the submissive, possibly forcing the submissive to assist her in reaching a climax, to really make the submissive yearn to enjoy that same feeling of release.

Keep in mind, the opposite can also be a form of punishment. Yes, as surprising as it sounds, allowing the submissive to have an orgasm can actually be punishment, when done in a certain way. The dominant may force the submissive to orgasm through stimulation the submissive doesn't find enjoyable. Or the submissive may be required to orgasm a certain number of times without any sort of foreplay or emotional interaction. The orgasms will probably not be very satisfying without any accompanying "play" activities. There is an endless variety of other punishments you can dream up for your submissive. Here are a few suggestions:

- Order the submissive to reach orgasm a certain number of times that day or week, without any assistance from you. This can be especially uncomfortable or embarrassing if it covers a period when the submissive will be at work or out in public.

- Make your submissive wear a chastity belt (available through BDSM sites and some adult stores). These are available for both men and women, but can be physically uncomfortable or even painful, so they are not for everyone.
- When you are out in public somewhere together—say, at a fancy restaurant—at some time during the evening, order your partner to take a sex toy into the bathroom and pleasure herself to orgasm without alerting anyone else who may enter the bathroom. To add an extra element of intrigue, tell her you will be timing her and may inflict another punishment if she takes too long to return.
- Make the submissive wear Ben Wa Balls, vibrating panties, clamps, or other items for a period of time while at an event (either alone or with you).
- Require the submissive to remain totally passive while you pleasure yourself with him or explore his body. He is not allowed to make any noise or react in any way.
- If your partner must go to work or run errands for the day, make sure she has a constant reminder of her punishment. For example, if your female submissive is shy or conservative, make her wear a revealing camisole or some trashy lingerie under her clothes.
- Get a temporary tattoo and make your submissive wear it to indicate he is "branded" as a bad boy (or girl).

Some Final Thoughts

Although punishment is a basic ingredient of a BDSM relationship, it is important to approach it from the right place. You never want to impart punishment when you are overly emotional or angry. Also, of course, you do not want to cause any serious harm to your partner.

Make sure your submissive knows that, although you may be displeased with her and need to punish her, you still care about her and love her. After the punishment is over, be sure to show your partner the affection and tenderness she deserves.

Also, remember that punishment is important, but so are rewards. You may want to establish a system in which the submissive can earn rewards. Perhaps he will receive a number of points for doing specific actions that please the dominant. This gives the submissive motivation to go out of his way to please the dominant.

Chapter 9

Role-Play and Fantasy

"Sex pleasure in woman is a kind of magic spell; it demands complete abandon; if words or movements oppose the magic of caresses, the spell is broken."

—Simone de Beauvoir

Role-playing and fantasies can be an important part of a healthy and satisfying sex life. These activities can be a way to add lots of fun and intrigue to any sexual relationship—but they tend to be particularly prominent in a BDSM arrangement. Many aspects of the BDSM lifestyle and the type of sex play it involves are based on or connected to fantasy and acting out certain roles.

For many people, the things they do as part of their BDSM play (or any type of sex play) are a way for them to shed their everyday personas and adopt whole new personalities, at least for a period of time. Role-playing lets you break free of your usual image and become someone completely different for a while—perhaps someone wild and bold, or if you prefer, someone shy and docile. So it only makes sense that people who enjoy BDSM activities would spend a lot of time engaging in role-playing and sharing—and possibly acting out—their fantasies with their partners.

Some people are reluctant to engage in role-playing at first. It may seem strange or embarrassing, or they may be afraid of revealing exactly what types of things turn them on. And yes, the first few times you try to act out different roles, it may be awkward and you may just end up sharing a lot of laughs with your partner. But hey, that's not a bad thing!

But chances are, once you become more comfortable and get into the groove, you will find you really enjoy these types of fun games. It is like playing a naughty adult version of the pretend games you enjoyed as a kid. Only here, there are no rules—you can pretty much do whatever turns you on, and indulge your imagination as well as your sexual urges.

The same thing goes with fantasies. Many people are often reluctant to share something so personal, and may be uncomfortable about revealing private thoughts that could be embarrassing or shocking. But if you and your partner have established a strong bond of trust, you should feel safe enough to open up in this way. And, of course, the feeling should be mutual. Make sure your partner feels comfortable enough to share his or her private thoughts and fantasies with you, as well.

The most important things here—as with any BDSM activities or sexual behavior in general—is to feel safe, secure, and respected enough to reveal yourself, both physically and emotionally, without fear of being hurt, embarrassed, or judged.

Sharing Your Fantasies

Revealing your secret sexual fantasies can be very exciting. It can also help strengthen your intimate bond with your partner. Sharing such private thoughts can be scary, however. You may never have revealed these things to anyone before. Opening yourself up to your partner and exposing your innermost desires requires deep mutual trust, as we've already discussed.

It may help to set some ground rules, such as agreeing that neither of you will ever criticize or make fun of the other's fantasy, no matter how "silly" or shocking it may be. And, of course, you should always hold this information confidential. Never betray your partner's trust by disclosing her fantasies to anyone else.

If you are a bit hesitant and have trouble getting the ball rolling, try making a game out of it. As an icebreaker, you and your partner can start by coming up with a few prompts that might help. For example, you might start with something like, "I always wondered what it would feel like to . . ." Or "It really turned me on when I thought about . . ."

Things can get really exciting and move in an entirely new direction when you share something your partner might never have expected. Admitting you are turned on by something that seems totally out of character for you will be a sexy surprise for your partner—and might cause him to see you in a whole new light.

If you suspect your partner has a secret turn-on she has been reluctant or embarrassed to reveal, you might want to make things easier for her by mentioning something along the same lines that you have fantasized about. This will give your partner an opening to share her own similar fantasies—or perhaps something altogether different that you hadn't expected.

Remember there is a big difference between fantasy and reality. Just because you may find the thought or image of a particular activity arousing does not mean you actually want to carry out the scenario. For example, some people find it arousing to imagine having sex with a person of the same gender—but this does not necessarily mean they really want to engage in same-sex activities in real life. The same goes for fantasies involving group sex.

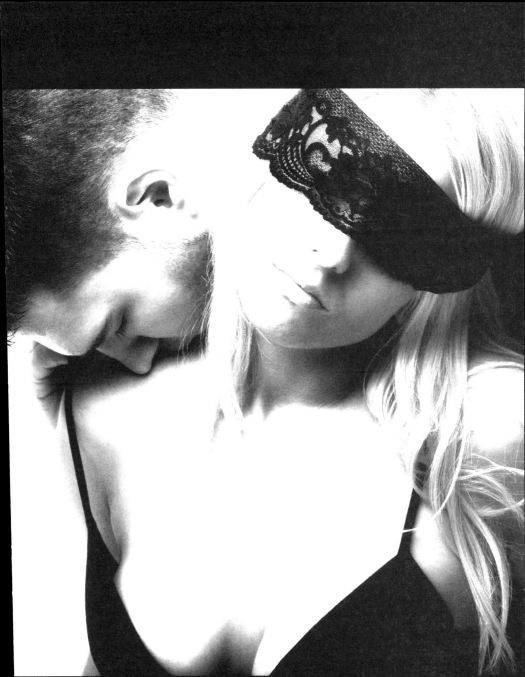

Some people may be reluctant to disclose these types of fantasies for fear their partners will then pressure them to carry out the actual activities, so it is important for you to reassure your partner that you can treat his fantasies as exactly that: fantasies that will not necessarily translate into real-life action.

Some middle ground exists, though. For example, if your partner fantasizes about group sex but does not actually want to engage in it, you might suggest watching an adult film involving group sex or visiting some online voyeuristic sites that allow you to watch group sex in action. Or if you are comfortable with the idea, considering visiting a club that allows you to just watch others in action.

 Kinky Tip

An ABC News survey found young people are more likely to discuss fantasies with partners than older couples—71 percent of those ages eighteen to twenty-nine did, compared with only 49 percent of those forty to forty-nine. In addition, 21 percent of respondents fantasized about a threesome, whereas 10 percent fantasized about having sex at work. Surprisingly, 30 percent fantasized about cheating on their partners, although only half of those admitted to actually being unfaithful.

One common type of fantasy couples share involves revealing the famous people who turn them on. This is something you can incorporate into your sex play in a fun way. Perhaps your partner can do an imitation of your celeb crush while you are playing. Or you could watch some hot footage of the star and use it as sort of a porn flick while you are having sex. It will be *almost* like having a threesome with your celebrity turn-on.

You might even jokingly come up with a "free pass" list. This is a list of, say, five famous people that your partner gives you permission to get physical with, should you ever have the chance. (However, if you work in an industry that actually gives you the opportunity to interact with famous people, you might want to proceed with caution in creating this list, or establish additional ground rules.)

Which brings us to a word of warning. There are no hard-and-fast rules about fantasy sharing, and you should feel comfortable enough to be open and honest. However, one area where you might want to tread carefully is admitting you fantasize about another person you and your partner know and interact with on a regular basis. Say, your boss. Or your partner's best friend. No matter how much your partner assures you he is okay with knowing the information, it almost always ends up making things uncomfortable, and can also make your partner feel nervous and insecure when you are around that person.

Perhaps the one exception to that rule would be if you are open to (or already engage in) threesomes, and you suspect the person you have in mind would be into it, too—and is someone your partner would be interested in playing with. Even so, proceed with extreme caution because these types of situations—no matter how well-intended they start out—have a strong risk of becoming very messy.

Basic Role-Playing

Many couples enjoy the sexy fun of role-playing. Role-playing can take many forms, as can the actual roles you decide to act out. It may just mean that you and your partner have a running storyline or dialogue (in your pretend roles) as you are acting out your fantasies.

On the other hand, you might choose to make a big production out of it, even going so far as to get props and dress up in costumes. Let your imagination run wild! This is a great way to add fun (and perhaps some laughs) to your sex play. It can also invoke a sense of mystery and spontaneity, because you will be adopting roles that are probably very different from the usual selves you're both familiar with.

As with fantasies, there are really no rules with role-playing. You can act out any type of characters or scenarios you want (assuming you and your partner are both okay with it, of course). Again, this should be a judgment-free environment, so don't worry about looking silly.

 Kinky Tip

Got a great idea for a role-playing scenario and want to surprise your partner? Leave a few props or accessories around, or some clues as to what scenario you may be acting out. How about sending a package to him at work with a few hints. This will heighten the suspense and jumpstart your partner's imagination—he'll be hot all day thinking about what's going to happen later. You might even decide to include these in your game.

If you are just broaching the idea of BDSM and haven't actually reached the point of becoming a dominant or submissive yet, this is your perfect chance to try it out. Pick the role of either dominant or submissive and act it out—really get into it and be convincing—and see how it feels. You and your partner can take turns switching roles, to see which one of you feels most comfortable in which role.

One great thing about role-playing is it gives you permission to act in a way that may be totally unlike your everyday behavior. This is the perfect excuse to let that inner tigress finally come out to roar! If you tend to be on the shy side, take advantage of the opportunity to be bold and aggressive. You don't need to be embarrassed. After all, it's not you—it's just a character you are portraying.

Part of the fun of role-playing is coming up with your own creative scenarios. But if you are just starting out or can't seem to think of any ideas, there are some tried-and-true standard setups that many couples have enjoyed. Take these as starting points, and put your own sexy twist on them!

Athlete and Cheerleader

You may never have had the faintest hope of making it to the big leagues—or even the junior varsity squad—but now you have the chance to live out your dreams of being a "big baller." Maybe your partner can even create a special cheer just for you. And if you have always thought cheerleaders were snobby, this is your chance to put one in her place. The best part: you are virtually guaranteed to score!

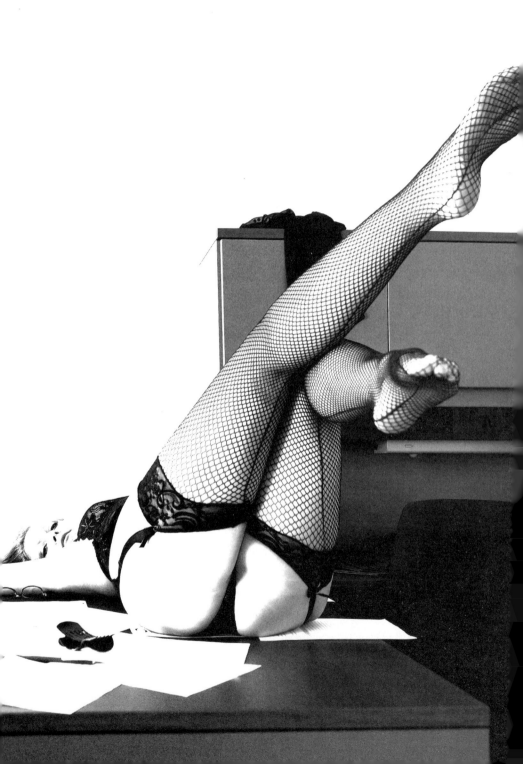

Steward/Stewardess and Passenger or Pilot

Give new meaning to the term "cabin service." Having a stewardess at your service will make you feel like you are going first class all the way and you may find yourself in the "fully upright position" way before takeoff. If you can't join the Mile High Club in real life, this can be an exciting alternative. Or you can be the master of your cockpit and show the sexy steward or stewardess exactly what you mean by "captain's orders."

Nurse and Patient or Doctor and Nurse

The best part about this scenario is, if you are the patient, all you have to do is lie in bed and enjoy the tender loving care of your knockout nurse. If you are really lucky, maybe she will give you a sponge bath. Or you can play doctor and nurse, and sneak off for a quickie in the supply closet. Or give each other examinations.

Boss and Secretary

The "boss" can chase the "secretary" around the desk, or come up with some creative types of sexual harassment. In a real office environment, it would be totally inappropriate to make your secretary service you orally from under the desk while you are on a conference call, or to make her answer your phone while she straddles you in the nude. Fortunately, this is your fantasy office, where anything goes.

Rich Lady and Pool Boy

You are a strapping young man just trying to make a living in the hot sweaty sun—which forces you to take off your shirt, of course. Suddenly you spot the rich lady of the house, strutting around poolside in her skimpy bathing suit. The pool boy can offer to assist the lady of the house in applying her sun lotion—or perhaps she will decide to do some topless sunbathing.

Repairman and Lonely Housewife

This is the premise of many a classic porn flick. The virile young contractor arrives to fix the leaky roof—only to be greeted by the housewife in her revealing negligee. She is bored and lonely at home by herself all day and it has been way too long since she has been satisfied by a man. The repairman's job is to show her exactly what she has been missing—but he has to finish the job before her husband gets home.

Teacher's Pet

In real life, of course, any sexual contact between teacher and student would be a no-no. But in your fantasy world, there is no such taboo (well, maybe there is, but you are allowed to do it anyway—that's what makes it so exciting). Let's see how far the student is willing to go to earn that A. She shouldn't be too shocked if her teacher bends her over the desk, entering her from behind. For added effect, the "student" could sport some cute pigtails that bounce up and down as the thrusting picks up speed.

Cop and Criminal

You can start things off with a thorough frisking, but most likely a strip search will be necessary at some point. And this is the perfect time to break out those handcuffs! For the woman playing the role of the criminal, you know what to do (hint: think of Sharon Stone in *Basic Instinct*).

Getting More Creative

Already tried the basics? Looking for something new and different? Let your imagination run wild. Try taking some of the standards and shaking them up—perhaps by switching gender roles or adding an unexpected twist. You can also browse adult message boards and see what role-playing games other couples have tried. You might be inspired. Here are a few creative ideas to help get you started:

Rock Star and Groupie

You are the devoted female fan who would do anything —yes, anything—to get close to your favorite rock star. Even if you have to flash your ass to every bodyguard and roadie backstage, you are determined to succeed in your mission. And it works—you finally make it onto the tour bus, where you can get up close and personal with the star himself. He offers to give you a tour of the bus, especially the bedroom, where you will have a chance to earn a VIP pass. But why should the guys have all the fun? Switch things up, with the female partner as the rock star and the male partner as the groupie.

Sworn Enemies

You (okay, your characters) aren't in love with each other. You don't even like each other. And yet can't deny the electric sexual energy between the two of you, and once you hit the sheets, you realize you have amazing physical chemistry. Can you put up with each other in order to have mind-blowing sex?

Tarzan and Jane

If you can manage to locate a loincloth (or make one yourself) that would be perfect. If not, any kind of jungle-print bikini briefs will do. This is your chance to act totally uncivilized and follow your most basic instincts. The phrase "fucking like animals" is a perfect fit here. And if you want to let loose with a "Tarzan yell" at the peak of excitement, feel free.

Cowboy and City Girl

Cowboys know how to get dirty. They also know a lot about mounting and riding. City girls don't know much about rodeos, but they do know how to look sexy in high heels. They also really appreciate how great a man's ass can look in a pair of tight, well-worn jeans or chaps

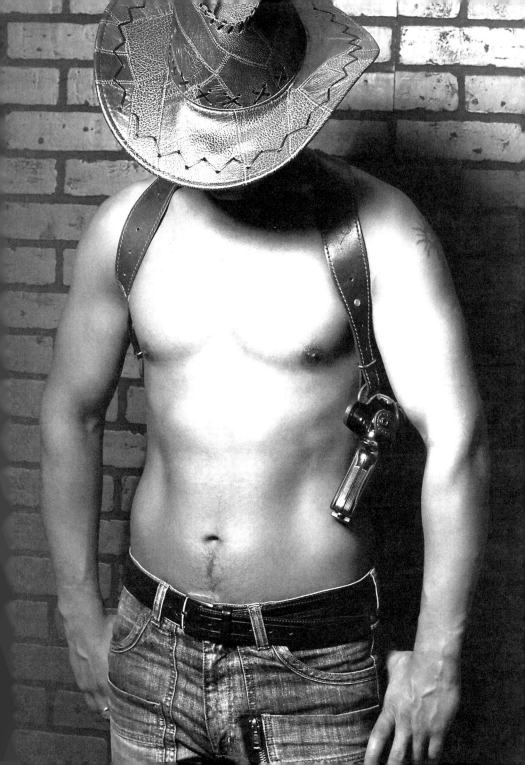

that leave his butt and other delicious parts totally bare. This is also the perfect opportunity to bring out your lasso and hogtie the city slicker.

Librarian and Frat Boy

She's a mousy, uptight librarian badly in need of a man who can loosen that bun of hers and let her hair tumble down. He's a laid-back frat boy, always ready for a good time. The only question is, will you get busy in the frat house or in one of the cramped aisles of the library's reference section?

Prostitute and Client

You and your partner can pretend to be Julia Roberts and Richard Gere in *Pretty Woman*—or a much dirtier, raunchier pair of temporary lovers. The plot of this story is totally up to you to decide—as is your "asking price."

Exhibitionist and Voyeur

One of you gets to strut your stuff (naked, of course) while the other watches from some hidden vantage point. The exhibitionist can take advantage of the opportunity to put on a really good show for her secret admirer, perhaps even going out of her way to tease the Peeping Tom.

Scientist and Lab Rat

One of you is the serious and nerdy scientist, the other is the test subject. The scientist wants to research the human anatomy, or perhaps test certain sexual reactions. So she conducts sexual experiments and probes in all sorts of areas, carefully observing the results and noting the responses of her subject.

Young Man and Seductive Cougar

Think *The Graduate* or *American Pie*. There is a reason "cougars" are so popular today. These experienced ladies have lots of tricks to teach younger men—and they get a thrill out of breaking in wide-eyed innocents. They also appreciate the young men's stamina that older guys often lack. It's up to the young man to shower the woman with appreciation.

Bodyguard and Celebrity

Make sure your partner is clear about the fact that his or her duty is to guard your body, as closely as necessary. You are sick of hangers-on and star-fuckers just using you and bragging to their friends. You need someone you can trust with your personal safety and well-being—and any other personal needs you may have.

Good Girl and Bad Boy, or Vice Versa

This is a classic "opposites attract" pairing. It usually ends up with the bad boy corrupting the good girl—or the girl shedding her Goody Two-Shoes skin. Think Olivia Newton-John in *Grease*. Or you could turn it around and make the good girl the seducer, like Molly Ringwald pouncing on Judd Nelson in *The Breakfast Club*.

Prison Guard and Female Inmate

A girl can get awfully lonely, going without the company of a man for so long. See if you can earn some privileges for "good behavior." You can help your guard get in the mood by sharing highlights of all the girl-on-girl action you've been having with the other inmates. Guard: don't forget the body cavity search.

Political Leader and Intern

You can probably guess what notorious encounter inspired this one. Service your partner while he is on the phone, seated at a desk. Throw in the cigar-related move, too, if you like.

Bolder Games

After you've had fun playing these games together, you might be feeling a bit more brave or daring. It's time to up the ante. Here are a few bolder games you can try—or use as starting points for your own racy scenarios.

Role-Play Together in Public

Come up with a scenario and give each other assignments before you head out into the world. One of you could try to pick up the other in a bar, or you can pretend to be strangers who decide to have a rendezvous on a train. Use your imagination. The knowledge that you might be turning on other people who are watching will make things even more exciting.

Be Online Exhibitionists

Lots of people get turned on by the idea of being watched while they're going at it. Find websites where couples can broadcast their sexual romps for viewers to see and enjoy. Warning: this is risky, as you are putting yourself out there for the entire world to see and you never know where the footage can end up. But if the thought really excites you, try it while you are both wearing masks, hoods, or something else that obscures your faces. Or position the camera (and your bodies) so that you are only visible from the neck down.

Be a Swinger, Online at Least

Join a swingers' message board. Nobody will know whether you are actually a swinger. In fact, this can be a great way to "try out" the

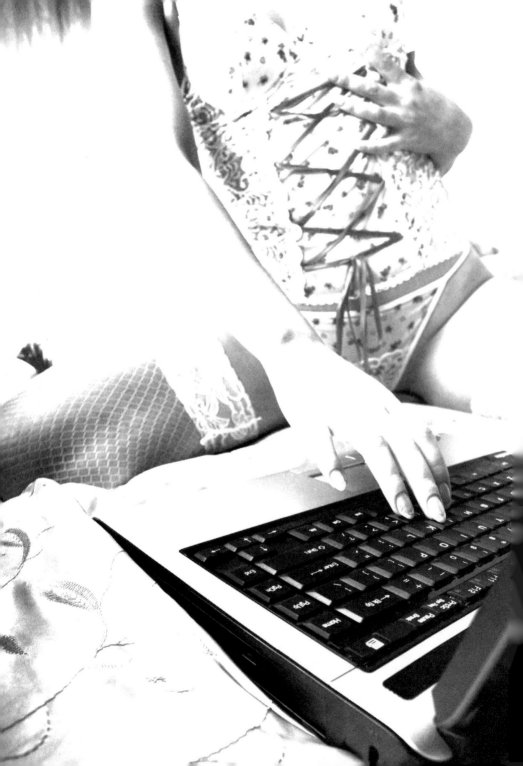

lifestyle, even if you aren't brave enough to actually do it. On many forums, you can read tales of exploits from actual swingers. In some cases, they will even post pictures or videos. Enjoying these with your partner can serve as a very exciting form of foreplay.

Phone Sex and Cyber Sex

If you get turned on by the idea of watching your partner have sex with someone else, but don't want an open relationship, you can allow her—assuming she is willing—to engage in phone sex or cybersex with someone online while you watch. You can pleasure yourself while watching the action, or join in and assist your partner in reaching a climax. Obviously, you'll want to take all necessary precautions to ensure your privacy and safety.

Toys and Props

What fun are games if you don't have toys to use for them? Toys are an essential ingredient for fun sex play. Most likely, you already have some sex toys in your drawer or treasure chest. But you may want to add some toys just for the purpose of acting out your role-playing scenarios.

Aside from actual sex toys, many other items can be used to spice up your sex life. We have already discussed ways in which you can use dusters, scarves, neckties, and other common household items. You may choose to use props that compliment your particular sexual fantasy. For example, if you want to enact a student and teacher fantasy scenario, consider adding props such as a desk and textbooks. And you thought chemistry couldn't be sexy! You might keep a paddle or cane nearby and punish the errant student with a spanking.

You don't always have to plan your scenario to the letter—it can be fun to try an improv approach. Have a grab bag or drawer with a random assortment of toys and props. Pick a few without looking—this is a great chance to break out that blindfold. Then come up with some sort of sexy scenario that incorporates the items you have chosen.

With a little creativity and imagination, you can devise ways to incorporate "mainstream" items—meaning things not designed with sex in mind, such as pancake turners—as props in your sex play. One up side is that you can buy these items at many locations, not just sex shops, and you won't be embarrassed if friends or relatives spot these innocent-looking items in your home.

If you want to go to the other end of the spectrum, you could choose something obvious, say, a sex swing where your submissive will be perched in the nude while you enjoy the view. Of course, this might be better to install in your playroom or a private area of the home, unless you don't care what visitors think.

Clothing, too, is often used as a sex life enhancer. Clothing—especially the right clothing—can sometimes be sexier than nudity. Obviously, lingerie and other sexy garments can be very effective. But try thinking outside the box—figure out ways to make work clothes or business attire provocative. For example, you can cut strategic

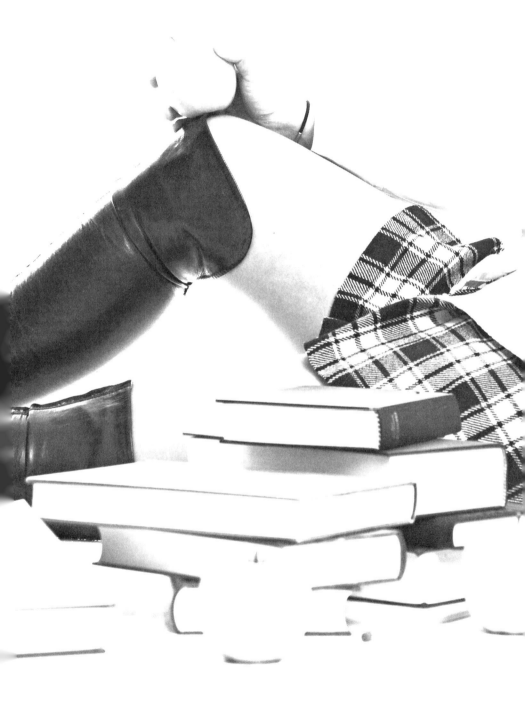

openings into your work overalls or add some sexy accessories to your office ensemble.

For some people, the sight and sound of clothing being ripped off in a passionate fury can be a turn-on. Pick up some inexpensive items at a thrift store or yard sale that you can tear off each other's bodies.

How about buying a pair of personalized underwear to delight your partner? Or if you are the dominant, buy undies with your name on them for your submissive to wear. This clearly announces that the body parts belong to the owner whose name they bear.

Here are some costumes that should be relatively easy to find and can greatly enhance your role-playing and fantasy activities.

- Cheerleader: If you weren't a cheerleader, you can usually find these uniforms at a Halloween store or costume shop.
- Nurse: Try a secondhand store. You can also buy scrubs just about anywhere.
- Rock star: Have you seen the way rock stars dress these days? Take the grungiest thing from the bottom of your closet, add some ripped jeans with holes in strategic places and maybe some costume jewelry, and you're good to go. Or if your fantasy star comes from an earlier period, say the psychedelic sixties or disco era, you can probably find appropriate garb online or at a shop that specializes in retro clothing.
- Doctor: Look for scrubs, or try to find a white coat at a medical supply store or uniform shop. A stethoscope can be a nice accessory.
- Athlete: Sporting goods stores are good places to find jerseys and other athletic attire.

- Hooker/stripper: This one is easy, just look for the trashiest store around, or head to the largest lingerie shop in the area.
- Schoolgirl: Scour thrift stores for school uniforms, or just wear a really short skirt and knee-high socks.
- Dominatrix: You will probably need to visit an adult store or BDSM website to find what you need.

Chapter 10

Taking the Kink Out of the Bedroom

"There is more to sex appeal than just measurements. I don't need a bedroom to prove my womanliness. I can convey just as much sex appeal, picking apples off a tree or standing in the rain."

—Audrey Hepburn

Not all of your "bedroom fun" has to take place in the bedroom—or your playroom, for that matter. There are lots of ways you and your partner can have fun outside of the house. In fact, it can often be very exciting to have sex in a new location. A change of scenery can make things feel new and different. Plus, different locations often provide options for creative positions and other elements that can make the experience thrilling.

So where can you go? Pretty much anywhere you want! Think about all the different locations you have access to or visit on a regular basis. Many people love the sensory experience of the great outdoors. With enough creativity and determination, you can probably find a way to enjoy some sex play in just about any location.

Of course, this can be riskier or more difficult to pull off in some places than others. For example, if for some reason you get turned on at the thought of getting it on in a jail cell, that might be a challenge. But most likely, the location you choose won't be quite as tough—and won't require you to break the law in order to get access.

If you have pretty much limited your sex play to your bedroom or playroom up until this time, you might want to start out with something relatively safe, such as a hotel room in a romantic location. Or pick a quiet and isolated spot outdoors where you are unlikely to get caught.

Many locations involve the risk of getting caught, and possibly getting in trouble—which for some people is a real rush and makes the encounter more exciting. In some cases, there may also be the chance that other people will see you—which again may be a turn-on, especially if you have some exhibitionist tendencies.

A great thing about expanding your sexual horizons, geographically speaking, is that there is really no end to the possibilities. You can pick a popular tourist spot, a foreign location, a scenic outdoor site, a public building—you name it. Want to be near the ocean? Head to the beach. Like the idea of someone watching? Pick a public location where you might be seen. Whatever you are craving, you can probably think of a location that will satisfy your urges, and provide a memorable experience for you and your partner.

If you have gotten into a rut or are seeking a way to add some zing to your sexual exploits, it may be time to take your show on the road.

Foreplay in Public

Public displays of affection aren't just romantic. They can also be very erotic. Many people like the idea of being watched while they are having sex. And if you aren't quite comfortable having actual intercourse with an audience, public foreplay can be the next best thing. It still gives you a taste of being an exhibitionist, without quite so much exposure.

Exactly how far you go in public and which location(s) you select for this adventure are totally up to you. It will depend on your comfort level, and the particular place you choose. Perhaps you will just have a make-out session at the movies. Or maybe you will feel up your partner's leg on the subway. If you are more daring, you could attempt something bolder. You will probably find that once you start engaging

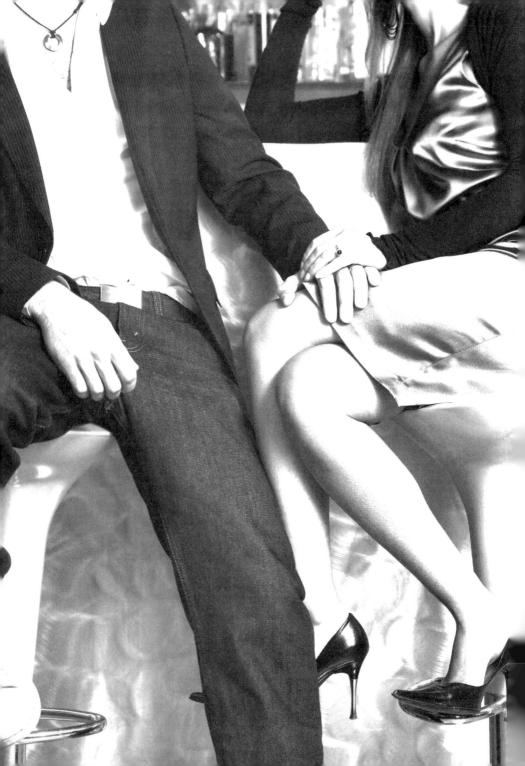

in foreplay in public, it's kind of a rush and you'll feel the urge to push the boundaries further next time.

Don't be surprised if you are constantly trying to outdo your last adventure in public. But that can be fun. You and your partner can take turns trying to raise the stakes and come up with exciting new things you can try in public. If you need inspiration, here are a few ideas:

- Find love in an elevator. This can involve several challenges, the first of which is getting an elevator all to yourselves (unless of course you want to be watched). You'll also have a built-in time restriction. You are pretty much limited to a quickie unless you hit the "stop" button.
- Make out at the movies. Yes, we know you probably watch most of your flicks at home in DVD format. But this is an old classic for a good reason. You will enjoy making your own movie magic. This is probably best attempted in a movie intended for an adult audience.
- Get wild while washing your car. You are already probably wet and soapy—it's a natural turn-on. Just be sure to head inside when things reach a graphic point if you are in full view of your neighbors.

Other People's Homes

Sometimes getting out of your own home—even if it just means going to someone else's—can provide enough of a change of scenery to make

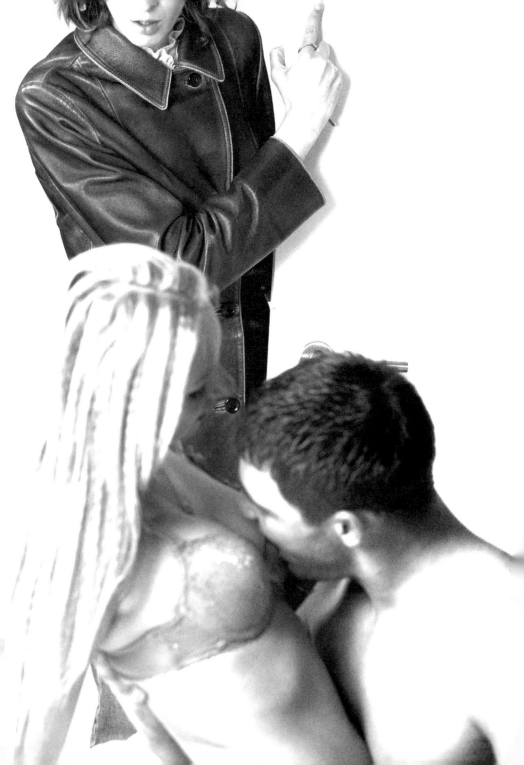

things seem new. The challenge, of course, is to get access to someone else's home and find a private area where you can play.

If you will be attending a party, look for an opportunity to enjoy a quickie. Take your partner by surprise by sliding into the bathroom. Or find an empty guestroom. Be prepared for some judgmental looks if other guests see you coming out looking flustered or disheveled.

If you will be going back to your childhood home for a visit, find a way to sneak in some sex. The idea of having sex in your childhood bedroom is exciting to some people, creepy to others. If it's a turn-on for you, figure out a way to escape the parents and get some privacy. You can pretend you are a teenager again and have snuck off for a forbidden make-out session while hoping your parents don't barge in.

Want to get it on in a really awesome house? Offer to housesit for some wealthy friends. Or ask a real estate agent to find you a furnished penthouse to rent for the weekend. You can also do this yourself online through one of the large vacation rental sites. Hire a caterer to cook and serve your meals, and enlist a pair of masseurs to give you and your partner a couple's massage.

Planes, Trains, and Automobiles

Vehicles are a very popular location for sex. In fact, for many people, their first sexual experience (perhaps even many of them) took place in a vehicle. This can bring back some memories for you—especially if you can manage to find a vehicle similar to one where you enjoyed some of your early encounters.

But you can also add an interesting twist by expanding your range and considering a variety of different types of vehicles. Think of exotic, strange, and unusual vehicles that might add a unique ambience (and possibly some sort of movement) to your encounter. Bonus points if it involves risk, or at least a sense of risk.

A basic idea to get you started is to have sex in a parked car. You will feel like a teenager again. For the full "flashback to high school" effect, down some cheap beer or wine coolers first and play some heavy metal music loudly in the background.

To increase the thrill and the risk, have sex in a parked car in a semipublic location. For example, a rest stop or the edge of a public park. The possibility of getting caught adds to the excitement. Just be sure to keep the doors locked and the keys in the ignition, should you need to make a quick getaway.

Another way to revisit the teenage years is to find your local lover's lane and go parking for a few hours. Make out in the car, doing as much groping and kissing as you can handle. But don't go all the way! This may help you rediscover the art of the kiss, and you'll remember why make-out sessions were such a thrill.

Have sex on top of a (nonmoving) car. Do it on the roof or hood of a car, and you will feel like you are in a music video or a bad porn flick. Just be warned: you may need to come up with a plausible explanation for that ass-shaped dent in the hood.

Do it on a motorcycle—one that isn't moving, of course. Be warned: a motorcycle is not the most comfortable surface on which to have sex,

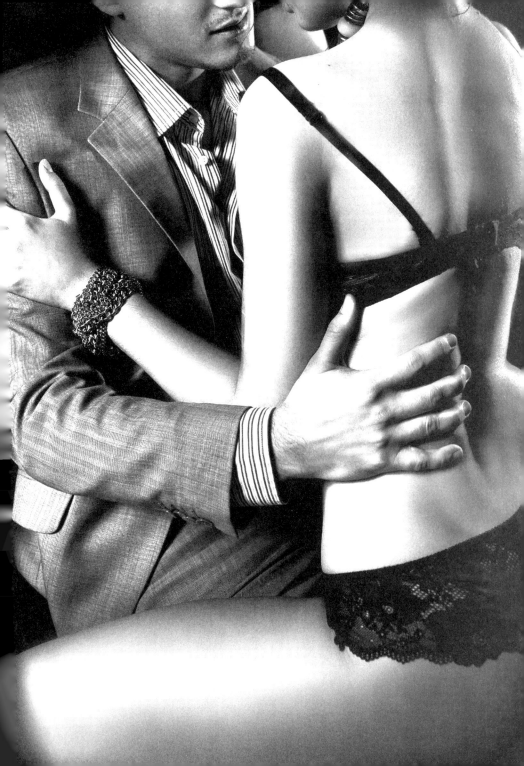

so this may be painful (and not in a good way); it also requires some flexibility.

Have sex in the back of a limo. This is something everyone should do at least once. If you didn't already check this off your list after the prom, now is your chance to rectify that situation. Having sex in the back of a limo will make you feel like a business tycoon or a celebrity. For bonus points, do it in the limo on your way to some big event. Not only will that start the evening with a bang, but you will share a naughty inside joke when you make your arrival and everyone wonders why you look so flushed.

A small boat is a great place to have sex, as it feels like a public area—and you also have the movement of the water. If you are susceptible to motion sickness, stay close to shore where the water should be relatively calm. Even better: if you have access to a yacht or can rent one for a few hours, you will get all the boat-sex benefits while also feeling like a big shot. Take advantage of the opportunity to christen the ship in a unique way.

Have sex in an expensive sports car. Frankly, many people feel this is overrated. Most sports cars are too tiny to allow for comfortable maneuvering. Plus, if it's a really expensive car, you or whoever owns it will probably freak out if you make a mess or damage anything. Still, it's cool to try this at least once—so consider renting a sports car and giving your partner a very special ride.

Have sex in the back of a pickup truck. Assuming that the tailgate is sturdy enough, one of you can lie in the back of the truck with your legs hanging down over the side while your partner services you.

Do it in the air. Yes, having sex in a plane is cliché. But if you have an opportunity to join the Mile High Club and don't jump on it, you will always regret it. To improve the experience, have sex in the first-class section. The accommodations are much nicer up there.

Have sex in the back of a van. Vans were made for sex, so don't let all that room go to waste.

Have sex in a Hummer. What's the appeal of sex in (or on) this vehicle? Well, let's see—it's big, it's bad—and hell, it's called a Hummer.

If you are going to have sex in a vehicle, add some of these items to really enhance the experience:

- Beaded seat covers
- Furry seat covers
- Leather seats
- Heated seats
- Throbbing sound system

Sex Outside

If you love the great outdoors, or just like the idea of being out in the open where there may be a risk that you will be discovered in a compromising position, think of locations outside where you and your partner may be able to have some fun.

This can be enjoyable because the environment adds some unique sensory elements, especially if there are seasonal influences. For example, being outside with exposed body parts in the fall or winter can give you chills in sensitive places, which can be very stimulating. Likewise, rain or snow—or the hot sun—can add sensations that enhance the experience and make it feel much different than it would if you were home in your bedroom.

Experiment with different types of surfaces and environmental backgrounds. This could involve anything from sand to mud, soft grass, a warm flat rock in the middle of a stream, or a roaring waterfall. Obviously, your options will depend on where you live and how far you are willing to travel. But most likely there are at least a few intriguing possibilities within a relatively short distance.

Sex on the beach is an obvious one. This is a classic, yet it is something surprisingly few people have actually done. Many beaches are deserted at night, and fairly dark too. The woman should wear a long, flowing skirt and leave her panties at home. Go out to a nice dinner, have some wine and flirt with each other, knowing what's coming for dessert. After dinner, stroll down to the beach and find a deserted spot.

Enjoy a sensual sunrise. Wake up before dawn, load blankets and coffee in the car, and drive to the beach. Watch the sun rise over the water. Bonus points if you can time your climax to coincide with the sun's first rays over the horizon.

Take a hike in the woods and look for a good spot to spread out a blanket and act like animals. Or look for a stream. With its gently rolling water, a stream is the perfect place for some outdoor fun. The flow of the water, the birds singing—it's straight out of a romance novel, but you get to make the ending as steamy as you want.

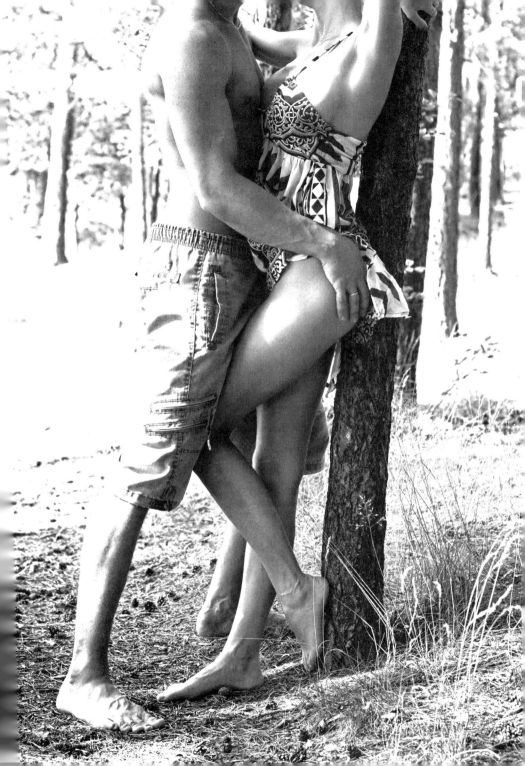

Want to stick to your own backyard? Have sex in a hammock. The swinging can provide a nice sensation—plus you'll be forced to lie very close together. Just be sure to test the hammock and make sure it is sturdy enough to hold the weight of two people.

If you have access to a relatively secluded body of water, go skinny-dipping. Whether you take a provocative plunge in the ocean or in a small private pool, a playful naked swim adds a sense of risk and adventure to any romantic getaway. Just be sure to leave your clothes in a safe, dry spot.

Try making some magic on a mountain. The view will be breath-taking (as will the thinner oxygen) so you will get a real adrenaline rush. Plus, you will most likely have the place to yourselves and can make as much noise as you want. Get a kick out of hearing your yells and moans echo all over the mountainside.

Get wild in a waterfall. It doesn't have to be a huge waterfall—you don't want to get swept away or pummeled by the water. As long as the water is flowing over the two of you, it will be an exciting rush.

Maybe you could put a sexy spin on a sporting event. If your partner is a sports nut, buy some tickets and accompany him to a game. Bring a blanket and do some scoring of your own. If your partner's team wins, treat him to a private victory celebration when you get home. You can add some special touches—say, dressing up in lingerie featuring the team colors. It will make the thrill of victory all the sweeter.

Give new meaning to a hole in one. Get busy on a golf course, per-haps while lying in the sun on the lush greens. Be sure to have your golf cart at the ready nearby in case you need to make a quick getaway. Oh, and watch out for wayward balls.

Risky or Unusual Places

Do you really want to ramp up the excitement and risk factor? Be bold and daring and try something really different or risky. You may need to give this some thought in order to come up with something especially good. You and your partner could make it a competition to see who can come up with the wildest idea.

If one of you is more hesitant, make it into a dare. Of course, the dominant could simply order the submissive to comply.

Here are some suggestions to get the ideas flowing:

- Sneak into work after hours and go at it in the boss's office. Unless he has a great sense of humor or a kinky side himself, you might have to look for another job if he ever finds out.
- Do a tour of famous landmarks—and make some sexy memories. Have a ball at Niagara Falls while the waves roar in the background. Go down on each other at the Grand Canyon. Indulge your horniness by the Hollywood sign. Rock the red-light district in Amsterdam (or a big city that's closer to home). Be creative. And don't forget to pick up a souvenir—it will always remind you of your adventure as wild tourists.
- Head to a motorcycle rally—ideally, a really big one like the annual gatherings in Daytona or Sturgis. Anything goes in this environment, and you will fit right in with the rest of the wild bikers. If you don't have a bike, borrow or rent one.
- Do it at the office, while on the job. This is easier to pull off if you and your partner work in the same place—or if you have your own

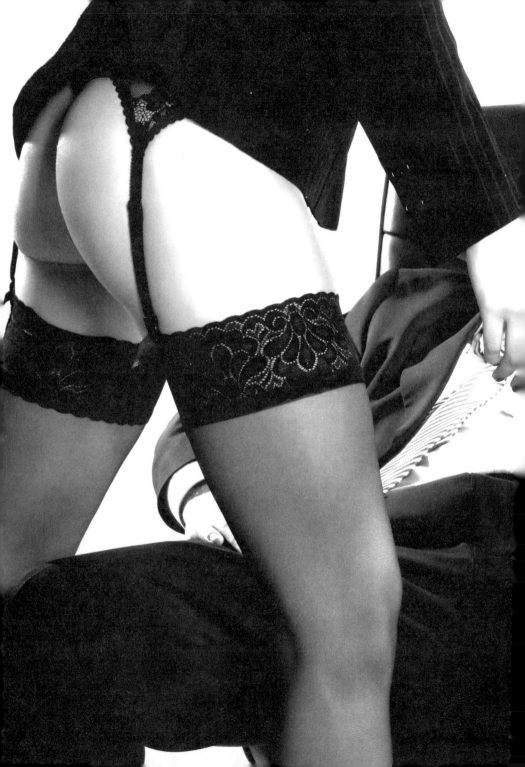

private office. It is much tougher to do if you work in a cubicle, or your workplace has a lot of security (or nosy coworkers who tend to work long hours).

- Have an encounter at a wedding. Wedding parties generally have loud music, lots of alcohol—and someone else is picking up the tab. The tricky part is finding a quiet, isolated spot where you won't be stumbled upon by the flower girl—or the minister.
- Other unusual places might include a hospital, cemetery (creepy for most people, but perhaps a turn-on for some), locker room, school (not while school is in session, obviously), hotel pool, sports stadium, playground, library, or the roof of a public building.

Conclusion

Hopefully this book has provided you with some tips and information that will help you feel more comfortable and excited about exploring the world of BDSM play with your partner. A healthy and satisfying sex life is an important ingredient for a good romantic relationship, and it is important to make your intimate relationship a priority.

Keeping your sex life fresh by trying new things will help prevent you from becoming bored or uninterested, and will add a new spark to your bedroom play!

Whether you are just taking baby steps into BDSM or are ready to jump in with gusto, the tips here will help guide you through this journey and help ensure your experience is as thrilling as possible.

Enjoy!

Index

Image Credits